# Specific Speech and Language Disorders in Children: Correlates, Characteristics and Outcomes

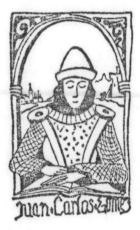

Juan Carlos Zumes

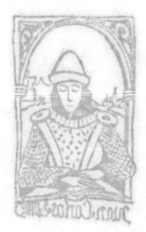

# Specific Speech and Language Disorders in Children: Correlates, Characteristics and Outcomes

**PAUL FLETCHER MA MPhil PhD**
*University of Reading, UK*

**DAVID HALL MB BS BSc FRCP**
*St George's Hospital and Medical School, London, UK*

With the assistance of Elizabeth Auger, Dorothy Bishop, Norma Corkish, Pamela Grunwell, Anthony Martin and Joy Stackhouse

W
Whurr Publishers
London

© AFASIC 1992
Ascociation For All Speech Impaired Children
347 Central Markets, Smithfield, London EC1A 9NH
First published 1992 by
Whurr Publishers Ltd
19B Compton Terrace, London N1 2UN, England

**British Library Cataloguing in Publication Data**

A catalogue record for this book is available from the
British Library

ISBN 1-870332-42-3

Printed and Bound in Great Britain by
Athenaeum Press Ltd., Newcastle upon Tyne.

# Opening address

## The President of the Czech and Slovak Federal Republic

A speech of mine called 'A Word About Words' seems to have given your director, Mrs Norma Corkish, the idea that I might be the right person to address the opening ceremony of your symposium which is dedicated to the problem of children who have difficulties with developing their powers of speech and language communication; the children who cannot use words in the way the rest of us take for granted.

I was thinking then, as I am thinking now, about the significance of words for human beings and for all their endeavours. But I also wonder why it is, that the same word can frequently mean many different things. Perhaps then, we should first give a thought to the concept of the word itself.

Is a word always and only a specific vibration of our vocal cords and, moreover, always an immutable symbol? Is a word always and only a particular mark on a piece of paper? And which of these two forms of the word is more important for us? Is a word, sounded with great difficulty by a human being with speech impairment, a less valuable word than some other? And is a word a lesser word when expressed by shape and movement of hands – the form and language of the deaf? I think a word, in any shape or form, is always only an imperfect tool for the process of expressing an idea.

Ideas are our most private wealth. They encompass not only the symbolic representations called words, but also our relationship with these words; a relationship which is shaped by our individual experience of life. Words, however, in their various shapes and forms, cannot be anything else but imperfect attempts at communicating ideas between human beings. And so the success of this communication depends much more on the extent of shared ideas between a speaker and a listener than on the actual words they use. After all, what makes us most importantly human is the life of our spirit; I mean our ability to create ideas, our ceaseless search for refining these ideas, and the subtle interaction of these ideas. I am convinced that this mysterious spiritual life, with its ideas and their interactions, is experienced not only by us, the ordinary people, but also by those who are very different from us. I sometimes even wonder who is the more impoverished by the communication barrier between us and those with impairment caused by speech and language disorders; a barrier which is also created by our inadequate symbolic representations, the words.

At this moment therefore, I think with great respect of you who are attempting to reduce the size of this barrier. I am sure that every one of your triumphs enriches both sides. I wish your association every success in its endeavours.

Vaclav Havel
Prague 20 February 1991

## PREZIDENT
## ČESKÉ A SLOVENSKÉ FEDERATIVNÍ REPUBLIKY

V Praze dne 20. února 1991

Dámy a pánové,

můj projev Slovo o slově přivedl Vaši ředitelku paní Norum Corkish k dojmu, že snad právě já bych mohl být tou správnou osobou,která by slavnostně zahájila Vaše Sympózium věnované problematice dětí, které nemohour rozvinout řeč pro těžká neurologická postižení. Které tedy nemohou používat slova v té podobě, kterou my ostatní považujeme za samozřejmou.

Zamýšlel jsem se tehdy nad významem slov pro lidské bytosti i pro veškeré jejich konání. Zamýšlel jsem se však i nad tím, že jedno a totéž slovo může znamenat různé věci. Měli bychom se možná zamyslet i nad samotným slovem Slovo.

Je slovem vždy jenom vlnění vzduchu rozechvělého našimi hlasivkami, a to ještě ve více či méně ustálen podobě? Je slovem vždy jenom jakási značka na papíře? A která z těchto dvou podob slova je pro nás důleži - tější? A je méně slovem zvuk vydaný s velikými obtížemi lidskou bytostí s poruchou řeči? Je snad méně slovem tvar a pohyb rukou - znak - znázornění neslyšícím? Slovo v jakékoliv podobě je vždy jenom nedokonalým vyjádřením pojmu. Pojem je naším nejsoukromějším vlastnictuvím. zahrnujícím nejen nálepku slova, ale i náš vztah k této nálepce daný celou naší dosavadní zkušeností. Slova ve svých různých podobách nemohou být ničím jiným, než nedokonalými pokusy o přenos pojmů mezi dvěma lidskými bytostmi a to, jak se tento přenos daří, záleží mnohem více na tom, do jaké míry se podobají pojmy mluvčího a posluchače. Lidské bytosti z nás přece dělá především náš život duševní, vytváření a neustálé upřesňování vlastních pojmů a jejich jemná interakce.

Jsem přesvědčen, že svůj tajemný duševní život se svými vlastními pojmy a jejich interakcemi prožívají i lidé, kteří se velice odlišují od nás - lidí běžných. A někdy se zamýšlím nad tím, kdo je vlastně více ochuzen komunikační bariérou, která pro nedokonalost nebo odlišnost přenašečů pojmů - slov, vzniká mezi námi a lidmi postiženými.

S hlubokou úctou myslím v tuto chv-li na Vás, kteří se ze všech svých sil snažíte právě o zmenšení této komunikační bariéry mezi námi a postiženými. Každý Váš úspěch přináší užitek oběma stranám. Přeji Vašemu jednání mnoho zdaru.

Váš

# Preface

After the success of its initial meeting in Reading in 1987, AFASIC (The Association for All Speech-Impaired Children) decided to organise a second International Symposium on Specific speech and language disorders in children. The conference was held at Harrogate, England, 26–31 May 1991. On each morning of the conference (on the final day into the afternoon), invited speakers from the different disciplines involved in language impairment presented plenary papers, together with the Symposium Keynote Address, given by Professor Sir Michael Rutter on the first evening of the conference. It is these papers that are brought together in this volume.

The main aim of the symposia that AFASIC has organised is to disseminate the latest research on language impairment in children to all those with a professional interest in these individuals. At this meeting, plenary papers were organised under topic headings similar to those of the first. The focus shifted through the week from external variables relevant for language impairment, to brain–behaviour relations, to the linguistic characterisation of language impairment, to outcome and management issues. Delegates were presented with an impressive range of information. In research terms 4 years, which was the period between the first and second symposia, is not a long time. It is perhaps a tribute to a dynamic field of inquiry that, even so, it is possible to highlight developments since the first meeting which could herald important new lines of research.

One of these developments arose out of the first symposium (as explained in Marcus Pembrey's paper). The investigation of a large family with a high incidence of language disorder affords the exciting possibility of, in time, being able to map the genetic mutation responsible for the speech and language impairment in the affected family members. The second area that is new since the first symposium is the cross-linguistic study of language impairment. Investigating the potentially distinct forms that language impairment may take in structurally different languages is likely to afford new insights into the mechanisms which are affected in the impaired individual. The third development reflected in some of the papers that follow is not so much an area of research as a changing perspective. There is a sense abroad that restricting enquiry to a narrowly conceived area of 'specific language impairment' may not be fruitful, either for research or for the affected individuals. The beginnings of a broader perspective in which (provided tight control is maintained over subject description) useful comparisons are made between different multidimensional profiles of language impairment across subject groups, are discernible here.

The production of a volume such as this would not have been possible without assistance. Caroline Roney once more organised the symposium with grace and efficiency. We are grateful to our contributors for their punctual present-ation of copy. Vanessa Hall made a considerable contribution to the difficult task of making consistent a variety of word-processing formats. To all involved, and particularly to our colleagues on the Symposium Committee, go our sincere thanks.

Paul Fletcher
David Hall

# Contents

# Contributors

**Dorothy M. Aram**
Case Western Reserve University and Rainbow Babies and Children's
Hospital, Cleveland, USA

**Dorothy V. M. Bishop**
MRC Applied Psychology Unit, Cambridge, UK

**Gina Conti-Ramsden**
University of Manchester, UK

**Paul Fletcher**
University of Reading, UK

**Pamela Grunwell**
Leicester Polytechnic and Birmingham Children's Hospital, UK

**David M.B. Hall**
St George's Hospital and Medical School, London UK

**Corinne Haynes**
Dawn House School (I CAN), Nottinghamshire, UK

**Patricia Howlin**
Institute of Psychiatry, London, UK

**Graeme D. Hutcheson**
University of Manchester, UK

**Judith R. Johnston**
University of British Columbia, Canada

**Laurence B. Leonard**
Purdue University, USA

**Lynn Mahwood**
Institute of Psychiatry, London, UK

**Ulrike Nettelbladt**
University of Lund, Sweden

**Marcus Pembrey**
Institute of Child Health, London, UK

**Katharine Perera**
University of Manchester, UK

**Richard Robinton**
Guy's Hospital, London, UK

**Sir Michael Rutter**
Institute of Psychiatry, London, UK

**David Skuse**
Institute of Child Health, London, UK

**Joy Stackhouse**
National Hospital's College of Speech Sciences, London, UK

**Jannet A. Wright**
National Hospital's College of Speech Sciences and the Institute of Education, London, UK

**Ann Zubrick**
University of Hong Kong

# Part I

# Factors Relevant to Language Impairment

# Chapter 1
# The biological
# basis of specific language
# impairment

DOROTHY V. M. BISHOP

The minimum requirements for language learning to take place are experience of language input, adequate sensory apparatus to perceive that input, and a brain which has the capacity to detect and learn the underlying structure of language when exposed to input. In addition, in order to produce speech as well as to understand language, there must be an articulatory apparatus which is capable of being programmed to produce speech sounds in a rapid and smooth sequence.

Children with specific language impairment (SLI) pose a puzzle. Their language acquisition is abnormal or delayed, yet they appear to have sufficient exposure to language input, normal capacity to perceive language, a brain which is adequate for learning in the non-verbal domain, and intact articulatory structures.

In this chapter I shall concentrate on possible biological bases of SLI. Many people have a stereotyped view of biological explanations, which are seen as rooted in a medical model that regards language disorder as a kind of disease which cannot be modified. If true, this would be a depressing picture for those concerned with remediation of SLI and it is perhaps not surprising that many people in those professions prefer explanations in terms of factors such as the home language environment. In this chapter I shall argue that biological factors are important and cannot be ignored, but at the same time I would stress that it is unrealistic to adopt a polarised view which treats biological and environmental approaches as alternatives. The causes of specific language impairment are likely to be multifactorial. Two factors that in isolation have no effect on verbal development may in combination lead to disruption of language acquisition. The combination of a non-optimal environment and a constitutional predisposition to language delay may be required to produce language disorder. Another point to stress is that the discovery of a biological basis to a disorder does not entail therapeutic nihilism. An environmental variable which plays little part in the causation of disorder may assume importance in its treatment. For example, I do not believe that there is any good evidence that the home language environment plays a major role in causing SLI. Most children develop normal language despite wide variation in parental communicative behaviour, and it seems unlikely that lack of verbal stimulation is sufficient to cause major language difficulties in children, except in cases where the child is subject to severe neglect or isolation (Mogford and Bishop, 1988). However, this does not mean that the home environment is unimportant; indeed, if a child does have a language disorder, it may be particularly important to ensure that the environment is structured to facilitate language development. Finally, if we can understand the underlying physiological mechanism for disorder, we may ultimately be able to discover biochemical methods of treatment or prevention. One of the clearest examples of this is the disorder phenylketonuria, a genetically determined disorder which affects amino acid metabolism and leads to mental subnormality if untreated. Once the biochemical nature of the disorder was understood it became possible to treat affected children by a restricted diet, with consequent dramatic improvements in intelligence (see Hay, 1985, for a review).

**Early Brain Damage**

The majority of children with SLI have no objective evidence of brain damage (Robinson, 1987; Haynes and Naidoo, 1991). Most have unremarkable neurological histories and no hard neurological signs. Disturbances of the electrical activity of the brain, as measured by electroencephalography, do characterise a minority of children with severe comprehension problems and the clinical picture of acquired epileptic aphasia, but in most cases no clear abnormality is found. Studies using modern techniques of brain imaging with SLI children are very rare. Computed tomography (CT) involves exposure to small amounts of radiation and many would argue that its use with children is not justified in research studies. Two studies which used CT scanning with SLI children without additional neurological handicaps were carried out by Rosenberger and Hier (1980) and Harcherik et al. (1985). Neither study found any structural lesions associated with SLI. An alternative procedure which is considerably more expensive but gives much higher resolution is magnetic resonance imaging (MRI). This procedure carries no known medical risk, but involves the child lying still inside an enclosed space in a noisy machine for a period of around 45 minutes. A controlled study using blind analysis of MRI with carefully selected SLI children was recently conducted by Jernigan et al. (1992). They found no evidence of structural brain damage in this sample, but, in common with Rosenberger and Hier, they did describe some differences from control children in terms of the relative size of different brain areas. Possible causes of such differences will be discussed in the next section.

Do these negative findings mean that we can rule out explanations in terms of early brain damage? The answer is not entirely, because not all forms of brain damage are detected by modern imaging techniques. Premature children of low birth weight commonly suffer from bleeding into the lateral ventricles of the brain (intraventricular haemorrhage, IVH). This can be detected in newborn children using ultrasound, but may no longer be evident after a few months or years, although there is an increased risk of developmental problems later in life. This raises the possibility that SLI may be caused by a 'hidden' brain lesion acquired around the time of birth. However, there are several arguments against this kind of explanation.

First of all, studies of children known to have sustained early brain injury typically find that any cognitive impairment is fairly general, and there does not appear to be an increased incidence of language disorders in children with normal IQ. Rather, one finds that non-verbal as well as verbal cognitive abilities are depressed. One might wonder, though, whether such group data mask individual variation in the pattern of disorder. We know that in adults the type of cognitive deficit observed is dependent on the location of the lesion, and language difficulties are specifically associated with damage to left frontal and temporoparietal areas. However, in children, the picture is rather different, because there is plasticity of functional representation in the brain, so that another area can take over a function if damage is sustained early in life. Children who suffer unilateral lesions of the language areas of the left hemisphere in the first 1 or 2 years of life will develop language in the right hemisphere. There is some debate as to how far there are cognitive costs associated with such reorganisation, but there is general agreement that there are no striking language deficits observed in children who sustain left hemisphere lesions, provided the damage is acquired early enough, and there is an intact right hemisphere that can take over language functions (see Bishop, 1988, for a review).

Is there any kind of early brain damage, then, that does cause specific language impairment? We would expect language to be impaired in cases of bilateral brain damage, where the language areas of the left hemisphere were affected but there was little or no opportunity for the right hemisphere to take over language function. In a recent study, Bendersky and Lewis (1990) investigated language development at around 16 months of age in children who had sustained IVH around the time of birth. IVH is typically bilateral, but one side may be more affected than the other. They found that level of language development was related to the amount of left ventricular dilatation, but not related to right ventricular dilatation. This study is consistent with the view that bilateral damage that is more extensive on the left than the right side of the brain may put the child's language at particular risk. However, we must await further follow up of children from this study before we can establish how specific and persistent these language problems are. It may be that left sided damage leads to delay in initial language acquisition while reorganisation of functional representation in the brain takes place, with normal progress later on.

### Non-genetic Prenatal Influences

When we consider ways in which normal brain function can be impaired, the obvious factors to consider are those which can lead to permanent destruction of neural tissue: infection, trauma or disruption to the oxygen supply. Any of these factors operating around the time of birth will result in a permanent loss of brain cells, because neurons cannot regenerate to repair brain damage after this age. However, there are much more insidious influences that operate long before birth to influence brain function, by affecting the very way the brain develops. The embryonic brain is first evident at 3 weeks' gestation as a slab of cells which rolls into a hollow tube between 21 and 25 days gestation. New cells are formed by cell division; these migrate to new positions in the developing brain and become differentiated into neurons and glial cells. Although on superficial inspection, the brain appears fairly uniform in structure, through a microscope one can detect a wide range of different kinds of neuron, organised in a highly systematic way, with cells of particular types arranged throughout the cortex in columnar structures. The delicate processes whereby cells proliferate, differentiate and migrate to the appropriate location in the brain can be affected by a host of factors including viral infection, drugs in the maternal circulation, exposure to irradiation or toxic agents, and nutritional status of the mother. In rats, it has been shown that stress in the pregnant mother can influence brain development of the offspring, and it is plausible that this may also be true for humans. Destruction of brain cells while the brain is still developing can result in a brain which is structurally abnormal as new cells migrate to the affected area, leading to areas of 'misplaced' neurons. The consequences of such factors are critically dependent on timing, e.g. rubella can cause major impairments in the fetus if experienced during the first 3 months of pregnancy, but may have little or no impact later on. Although we know something of the impact of factors which cause major handicaps, such as rubella, we remain largely ignorant of the role of such prenatal influences in causing more subtle impairments of brain development.

In a recent and highly influential theory, Geschwind and Galaburda (1985) proposed that levels of testosterone in the fetal circulation might be important for language development. The course of development usually differs for the left and right hemispheres, with certain areas of the left side maturing ahead of the homologous areas on the right. Geschwind and Galaburda proposed that this process is retarded by high levels of testosterone, which can therefore lead to the brain developing more symmetrically. This, they suggested, can cause lack of cerebral lateralisation, left-handedness and speech and language disorders. There is a lack of direct evidence for such a mechanism, but it could serve to explain why a higher proportion of boys than girls are affected by developmental disorders involving speech, language and reading. How far is this a realistic explanation for specific language impairment? Testosterone is known to have major effects on sexual differentiation of the prenatal brain, but its role in influencing asymmetric brain development remains purely speculative. Studies of individuals with disorders which affect hormonal levels, such as adrenogenital syndrome, do not support the prediction that laterality and language competence depend on testosterone levels (Pennington et al., 1987). There is, however, mounting evidence that the brains of individuals with developmental disorders affecting language and literacy skills are less likely to show a normal pattern of morphological brain asymmetry. This has been shown in several studies using brain imaging in dyslexic individuals (e.g. Haslam et al., 1981; Rumsey et al., 1986), and in two studies of children with specific language difficulties (Rosenberger and Hier, 1980; Jernigan et al., 1992). Nevertheless, one must beware of equating structural symmetry with functional symmetry. There is remarkably little evidence to support the view that language-impaired children are less functionally lateralised than other children. Contrary to popular belief, there is little hard evidence for an excess of left- or mixed-handedness in such individuals, and studies using techniques such as dichotic listening find poor performance overall, but no indication that language is mediated bilaterally or by the right hemisphere. Bishop (1990), in a review of the literature, concluded that it seemed likely that language is mediated by a poorly developed left hemisphere, rather than there being atypical patterns of functional lateralisation in these children.

As we have seen, there is little hard evidence to implicate particular prenatal factors in the causation of specific language impairment. Nevertheless, it is important to be aware of how brain development can be influenced by factors which are neither genetic nor disease based. The testosterone theory makes many assumptions which are as yet unsupported by data, but it does draw attention to the need of any theory of aetiology of SLI to explain sex differences in the incidence of disorder.

## Sensory Input During Critical Period

Influences on brain development continue to operate after birth. Although humans are born with a full complement of brain cells, and cannot develop any more if these are damaged, considerable changes occur in the first years of life as enormous numbers of neuronal inter-connections develop. There is ample evidence from animal experiments that in order to develop normally the brain needs appropriate sensory input. Most work has been done on the visual system of the cat. For example, in normal animals, there are cells in the visual cortex which respond to binocular stimulation and are important for giving a sense of depth perception. If the young kitten has one eye temporarily occluded, then these cells do not develop, and the animal's depth perception will be permanently affected. This work, which has important implications for treatment of squint in humans, has been used to argue that there is a critical period in an animal's life, during which neuronal connections are normally formed, when lack of appropriate sensory experience will pro-duce lasting impairment, even if normal visual input is restored later.

It has been suggested that the concept of the critical period may have relevance for language development in human infants, and that tempo-rary impairment of normal hearing early in life will have long-term detri-mental consequences by influencing how the auditory perceptual system develops. This notion assumes importance when one recognises that a substantial proportion of children are affected at some point in the first 3 or 4 years of life by a form of middle-ear disease, secretory otitis media, which causes build-up of fluid in the middle ear, usually with associated conductive hearing loss. The disease often goes undetected, unless spe-cial techniques such as tympanometry are used to measure the function of the middle ear. Population surveys have found that 30–40% of chil-dren suffer from three or more episodes of otitis media in the first few years of life (Klein, 1986). If there is a critical period when the child must hear clearly to develop normal connectivity in the auditory system, then the impairment of hearing caused by otitis media could lead to long-term auditory perceptual problems, even after hearing has returned to normal. Secretory otitis media, then, could provide a plausible explana-tion for language disorders in children with apparently normal hearing. How far does the evidence support this explanation?

It might seem to be a relatively simple matter to answer this question by comparing the incidence of otitis media in children with language impairment and a control group. However, things are not so simple. Oti-tis media is a transient disorder, and is often undetected. It is widely believed that the critical period for development of auditory–verbal skills is in the first 2 years of life, before language disorder is evident. The most relevant question, therefore, is whether the child previously suffered from otitis media, rather than when the disorder is currently present. However, this kind of retrospective reporting is fraught with possible bias: in some cases, the child may have had otitis media without anyone recognising it; on the other hand parents of language-impaired children will be seeking for an explanation of their child's problems, and may therefore be more likely to remember episodes of ear disease. Another approach that is sometimes adopted is to compare rates of language disorder in children with recurrent otitis media and those with no history of ear disease. Indeed, it was early studies of this kind that first suggested a link between otitis media and language disorder. However, this method too is problematical. If we had two children with otitis media, one of whom was developing normally and the other had language difficulties, then it is more likely that the otitis media will be detected and treated in the second child, because investigation of hearing status, and treatment of any problems, is standard clinical practice when dealing with a child with language difficulties. Where the child is developing normally, there is no incentive to investigate hearing function in the first place, so otitis media may go undetected, and even if it is identified, a conservative approach to treatment is more likely to be adopted if the disorder is having no apparent ill effect on the child's development. In sum, one cannot regard children recruited through otolaryngology clinics as a random sample of individuals with middle-ear disease: there is likely to be over-representation of children with language difficulties.

The only way of avoiding such bias when assessing the effects of otitis media is to screen a whole population for middle-ear disease over a period of time, and then compare those who had repeated episodes of otitis media with those who did not in terms of language development. Only a few studies of this kind have been conducted, and results have been mixed. Lous and Fiellau-Nikolajsen (1984) found no effect on reading achievement of previous repeated episodes of otitis media, but more recently Lous (1990) has reported a significant association between recurrent otitis media and phonological impairments in 7-year-old children. Silva, Chalmers and Stewart (1986) found statistically significant deficits in reading ability of children with a history of middle-ear disease at age 5, but the effect was small and there was no excess of children with severe specific reading disability among those with positive histories of otitis (Share et al., 1986). Teele et al. (1984) found small but statistically significant deficits on language tests for children who had had otitis media for prolonged periods in the first few years of life. Friel-Patti et al. (1982) carefully monitored the hearing status of 35 babies during the first two years of life and found that 71.5% of those with recurrent otitis media had language scores 6 months or more below age level; Roberts et al. (1986), however, failed to replicate this finding. A more comprehensive study of 483 children by Friel-Patti and Finitzo (1990) found significant effects on language development of hearing loss associated with otitis media in the first 2 years of life, but these were small in magnitude and the authors stressed that they did not find clinically delayed language in otitis-prone children.

How is one to synthesise these conflicting findings? Bishop and Edmundson (1986) drew attention to two factors that seemed to be important in determining whether or not language deficits would be associated with otitis media. First, the child's hearing status at the time of assessment was important. In general, the strongest evidence for language deficits associated with otitis media is found in studies where children still have otitis media at the time of assessment. There is less support for the idea that a past history of otitis media leads to permanent language deficits in children who have since recovered. The second point made by Bishop and Edmundson was that the effects of otitis media might vary depending on whether other risk factors for language impairment were present. This notion was suggested by their finding that in a language-impaired sample, otitis media and perinatal hazard tended to co-occur, whereas they were independent in a control sample. This finding should be treated cautiously, given that data were based on retrospective parental reporting, and Haynes and Naidoo (1991) did not find any association between otitis media and perinatal risk factors in a sample of more severely language-impaired children studied by similar means. Nevertheless these data at least raise the possibility that the combination of otitis media and perinatal hazard might have more severe consequences than either factor in isolation. It is noteworthy that the study by Friel-Patti et al. (1982), which reported unusually strong links between otitis media and language impairment, was conducted with children most of whom were of low birth weight. A speculative explanation may be proposed for these findings in the light of the critical period hypothesis. The experimental work with animals indicates that the impact of sensory deprivation is crucially dependent on the state of maturity of the nervous system. Indeed, the same experimental manipulation applied to immature animals a given number of days after birth will have different effects on different species whose offspring are born at different stages of development. One wonders, therefore, whether premature babies may be particularly vulnerable to the adverse effects of otitis media because their nervous systems are less mature at the time of birth. Prospective studies should be undertaken to evaluate this possibility.

Bishop (1987), in a review of aetiological factors in SLI, concluded that otitis media was unlikely to be a major cause of SLI. Although some effects on language development had been demonstrated, these were generally very mild. Furthermore, there are a number of features of SLI that cannot readily be accounted for in terms of this causal hypothesis, especially the sex ratio and the association with motor impairment. Nevertheless, it was suggested that otitis media may assume importance in some cases where other risk factors are already operative, and it was suggested that future research should be directed towards looking for evidence of synergistic influences in the aetiology of SLI, rather than considering individual factors in isolation.

**Genetic Influences**

The past 5 years have seen an upsurge of interest in the possibility that genetic factors may play a part in the causation of a range of developmental disorders (Rutter et al., 1990a). Evidence for genetic factors has been documented for autism, stuttering and developmental reading disorders, although in none of these cases does there appear to be a straightforward mendelian pattern of inheritance. Recently, several published studies have noted that children with SLI have an unusually high rate of affected family members (Bishop and Edmundson, 1986; Neils and Aram, 1986; Robinson, 1987; Tallal, Ross and Curtiss, 1989; Tomblin, 1989; Haynes and Naidoo, 1991), and one case of an extended family with a dominant pattern of inheritance for language disorder has been described (Hurst et al., 1990).

Given that the evidence for familial association of language impairment is so strong, it is interesting to consider why there has been so little interest in genetic explanations in the past. One reason may have been that most research on normal development has concentrated on documenting how language acquisition is related to language input that the child receives, and this has led many people to tacitly assume that if a disorder runs in a family, this represents a kind of 'cultural transmission', whereby the child receives inadequate language input from parents and siblings, and so develops inadequate language too. This, however, seems increasingly unlikely in the face of evidence that most families contain a mixture of affected and unaffected individuals. If poor parental language caused language disorder, then we would expect all children to be affected to some extent. In addition, we know that language development is surprisingly resilient, and children whose parents produce very limited oral language (because they themselves are profoundly deaf) seem nevertheless to make good progress, provided they are exposed to about 5–10 hours per week of speech from hearing people (Schiff-Myers, 1988).

The current interest in genetic factors is to be welcomed, but a great deal of work needs to be done to establish just how important genetic factors are, whether they are involved in all types of developmental language disorder or just a few, and how genes operate to influence language development. It is important to recognise that the fact that a disorder runs in families does not prove that it is inherited: apart from the possibility of cultural transmission, as noted above, there are also other environmental influences shared by family members that might be causally implicated.

Rutter et al. (1990b) have reviewed research strategies that may be used to gain a clearer picture of genetic bases of developmental disorders. One way of investigating the role of genetic factors in causing a disorder is to compare concordance rates (i.e. the percentage of cases where both twins are affected) in monozygotic (MZ) and dizygotic (DZ) same-sex twin pairs. The logic of the approach is as follows: MZ twins are genetically identical, whereas DZ twins have on average 50% of their genes in common. In both cases, the twins are reared together in similar environments. If we assume that the similarity of the home environment is no greater for MZ than for DZ twins (see Plomin, Defries and McClearn, 1990), then the difference in concordance rates for MZ and DZ twin pairs provides an estimate of the role of genetic factors in causing the disorder. In 1989, I started recruiting subjects for a twin study of SLI. The study has a further year to run, and only preliminary findings can be reported, but a number of interesting points have emerged from the early data which, on the one hand, offer some support for a genetic basis of developmental disorders, but which also suggest that other, non-genetic influences are important.

There are several methodological difficulties in doing a study of twins. One is recruitment bias. If one recruits children through professional colleagues, then it is likely that disproportionate numbers of concordant twins will be referred, simply because two children with the same disorder stand out as distinctive. The ideal way of avoiding such bias altogether is by sampling a whole population of twins and identifying those with language disorder, but when studying a relatively rare condition this is likely to be impracticable. Rather, an approach was adopted which aimed to minimise recruitment bias by recruiting where possible directly via parents, using advertising in local newspapers across the UK. Parents were asked to volunteer for the study if they had twins of the same sex aged at least 7 years, where one or both twins had had speech therapy for language difficulties that were not due to mental or physical handicap. Adults with SLI were also encouraged to refer themselves directly to the study.

Using this approach, 106 twin pairs have been seen and given a non-verbal IQ test (Ravens Matrices; Raven, Court and Raven, 1977) and a battery of speech and language tests. These include The Test for Reception of Grammar, TROG (Bishop, 1973), the Sentence Repetition subtest from the Clinical Evaluation of Language Functions (CELF; Semel and Wiig, 1980), Renfrew Word Finding Vocabulary Scale (Renfrew, 1980) and the Verbal Comprehension subtest from the Wechsler Intelligence Scale for Children – Revised (Wechsler, 1974). Data have also been gathered on experimental procedures designed to elicit samples of narrative and conversational speech, and on articulatory proficiency, but these have not yet been fully analysed, so are not considered here. In addition, parents are asked to complete a detailed questionnaire about the twins' early medical and developmental history. Wherever possible, medical records and speech therapy reports are consulted to supplement this information. Zygosity was determined using a standard zygosity questionnaire (Nichols and Bilbro, 1966), which relies on similarities in physical characteristics, although genetic  fingerprinting was used wherever the questionnaire was inconclusive and where permission was obtained to take blood samples from the twins.

The preliminary data reported here include those twin pairs where zygosity was unambiguous and at least one twin met the following criteria for SLI: a non-verbal IQ of 85 or over; and a score below the 5th centile on at least one test of language functioning. In some cases, children's records gave clear evidence of previous speech and language problems, although they did not meet criteria for SLI when assessed. Provided that the disorder had persisted beyond 5 years of age, and the child had received at least two year's speech therapy and/or special education for it, these subjects were included as cases of past SLI. Children with physical impairments of the articulatory apparatus were excluded from consideration, as were those with sensorineural hearing loss. When assessing concordance between twins, it was noted that in many cases where twins were discordant for past or present SLI, the co-twin nevertheless was not developing normally. These cases included: mentally retarded children with non-verbal IQs below 70; 'spectrum' disorders, i.e. those with non-verbal IQs in the range 70–85, with language scores below the 5th centile; 'borderline' cases, i.e. those with IQs in the range 70–85 with normal language scores; and reading disabled, i.e. those with nonverbal IQs of 85 or above, who had severe problems with reading and/or spelling (scaled scores of 75 or below), but normal scores on language tests.

Before going further, it should be recognised that it has been argued that the twin study method may give misleading estimates of heritability for language disorders, because there is some evidence that twinning itself affects language development (Hay, 1985). On average, twins obtain scores on language tests significantly below the singleton mean, even though non-verbal ability is normal (see Mogford, 1988, for a review). The reasons for this language delay are unclear: it has been suggested that this is because of the way twinning affects mother–child interaction in the early years, when the caregiver's attention and resources must be divided between two children at the same developmental level. The tendency of twins to communicate with one another in 'twin language' has also been implicated, especially as an explanation for delay in phonological development. An alternative view is that twinning retards rate of prenatal growth. What is not clear is whether twins are at high risk of clinically significant language disorders, or whether their language development is simply somewhat slower than average. If twinning itself puts a child at risk for SLI, then heritability figures derived from twin studies will underestimate the genetic contribution to the disorder. In order to estimate this possibility further, I looked at the incidence of language difficulties in other family members of affected twins, and compared this to the incidence seen in a sample of singletons with SLI. The figures are shown in Table 1.1. There is no significant difference in the frequency of affected relatives in the two SLI samples, both of which have appreciably higher rates of affected relatives than a control sample. This is reassuring in suggesting that the importance of familial factors in causing SLI is not appreciably different in twins than in singletons. Family history is scored as positive when there is a first-degree relative with definite history of language impairment. It is appreciated that this index is crude and does not take into account family size, but it is used here to provide a preliminary comparison of singleton and control children with SLI assessed on a common scale.

Table 1.2 shows data for the 61 twin pairs where at least one member meets criteria for current or past SLI. This twin is designated the proband; the other is termed the co-twin. If both twins are affected, then coding of proband and co-twin is done at random. If one twin had current SLI and the other had past SLI, the twin with current SLI was designated the proband.

Separate tabulations were conducted for probands with current SLI

**Table 1.1** Family history of SLI[1]

|                      | n   | No  |      | Yes |      |
|----------------------|-----|-----|------|-----|------|
| Control singletons*  | 155 | 151 | (97) | 4   | (3)  |
| SLI singletons*      | 56  | 38  | (68) | 18  | (32) |
| SLI twins            | 55  | 43  | (78) | 12  | (22) |

*From Bishop and Edmundson (1986).

Values in parentheses are percentages.

[1]Family history is scored as positive when there is a first-degree relative with definite history of language impairment. It is appreciated that this index is crude and does not take into account family size, but it is used here to provide a preliminary comparison of singleton and control children with SLI assessed on a common scale.

**Table 1.2** Status of co-twins in relation to proband diagnosis

|  | Proband with current SLI | | Proband with past SLI | |
| --- | --- | --- | --- | --- |
|  | MZ twins | DZ twins | MZ twins | DZ twins |
| Co-twin (n) | 26 | 12 | 13 | 10 |
| Current SLI | 9 (35) | 4 (33) |  |  |
| Past SLI | 8 (31) | 1 (8) | 9 (69) | 2 (20) |
| Spectrum | 5 (19) | 1 (8) | 1 (8) | 0 |
| Borderline | 1 (3) | 2 (17) | 2 (15) | 0 |
| Mental handicap | 1 (3) | 2 (17) | 0 | 0 |
| Reading disability | 1 (3) | 2 (17) | 0 | 0 |
| Normal | 1 (3) | 0 | 1 (8) | 8 (80) |

Values in parentheses are percentages.

and those with past SLI. It is apparent that there is a substantial difference in concordance for MZ and DZ twins among those with past SLI but concordance for current SLI is no higher for MZ than for DZ twins.

Perhaps the most striking feature of these data is the very high rate of associated disorders among co-twins of both MZ and DZ probands with current SLI. Only one co-twin of a proband with current SLI is coded as 'normal'. In fact, when data from this child were examined, it was found that he had received speech therapy for one year – not sufficient to merit inclusion in the 'past SLI' group, but enough to cast doubt on his categorisation as 'normal'. In short, there was no cotwin of a proband affected with SLI whose development was entirely normal. Although the numbers are far too small for firm conclusions, there do appear to be closer similarities in the type of disorder seen in co-twins of affected MZ twins than in those of affected DZ twins. Low non-verbal ability, in most cases above the level of mental handicap but within the 'borderline' range was common in all co-twins, but MZ co-twins seemed more likely to have poor language, either at the time of assessment or in the past.

Conclusions from these data must be tentative, given the preliminary nature of the analysis and the small sample size, but it is interesting to speculate on their significance. One interpretation compatible with the findings would be that genetic factors are important in the aetiology of language delay which eventually resolves, but more persistent language difficulties may only be seen when additional adverse factors are experienced. It is interesting to note that a similar distinction was drawn by Byrne, Willerman and Ashmore (1974), who found that children with moderate levels of SLI had significantly more affected family members than those with more severe disorders. However, those with severe disorders had higher levels of perinatal and postnatal neurological risk factors. In a similar vein, those studying genetic factors in reading disability have suggested that heritability might be greater for younger children with reading disability than for older children, although large samples would be needed to provide an adequate test of this view (Wadsworth et al., 1989). One way of interpreting the data from Table 1.2 would be to argue that for persistent SLI to occur one needs both a genetic predisposition to language delay and additional adverse experiences. If these adverse circumstances are experienced by a child with no predisposition to SLI (as in some co-twins of DZ probands with SLI) then a wide range of types of disorder, including non-verbal as well as verbal impairments, may ensue. However, if the same circumstances are experienced by a child with a genetic predisposition to slow language development, then impaired language development, with or without concomitant non-verbal retardation, will be seen. The nature of the postulated 'adverse circumstances' remains highly speculative, but the very high concordance for disorder seen in DZ and MZ twins would suggest that we should look for experiences shared by both twins. Perinatal brain damage is an obvious candidate, as are the kinds of non-genetic prenatal influences on brain development considered above. It is hoped that future analyses of birth history records of a larger series of twins from this study will shed further light on the mechanisms whereby environmental and genetic factors conspire to produce language impairment.

## References

BENDERSKY, M. and LEWIS, M. (1990). Early language ability as a function of ventricular dilatation associated with intraventricular hemorrhage. *Developmental and Behavioral Pediatrics,* 11, 17–21.

BISHOP, D.V.M. (1973). *The Test for Reception of Grammar.* Published by the author at Department of Psychology, University of Manchester.

BISHOP, D.V.M. (1987). The causes of specific developmental language disorder ('developmental dysphasia'). *Journal of Child Psychology and Psychiatry,* 28, 1–8.

BISHOP, D.V.M. (1988). Language development after focal brain damage. In D. Bishop and K. Mogford (Eds). *Language Developmen in Exceptional Circumstances.* Edinburgh: Churchill Livingstone.

BISHOP, D. V. M. (1990). Handedness and Developmental Disorder. *Clinics in Developmental Medicine, 110.* London: MacKeith Press and Oxford: Blackwell Scientific.

BISHOP, D. V. M. and EDMUNDSON, A. (1986). Is Otilis media a major cause of specific developmental language disorders? *British Journal of Disorders of Communication,* 21, 321–338.

BYRNE, B., WILLERMAN, L. and ASHMORE, L. (1974). Severe and moderate language impairment: evidence for distinctive etiologies. *Behavior Genetics,* 4, 331–345.

FRIEL-PATTI, S., FINITZO-HIEBER, T., CONTI, G. and BROWN, K. C. (1982). Language delay in infants associated with middle ear disease and mild, fluctuating hearing impairment. *Pediatric Infectious Disease,* 1, 104–109.

FRIEL-PATTI, S. and FINITZO, T. (1990). Language learning in a prospective study of otitis media with effusion in the first two years of life. *Journal of Speech and Hearing Research,* 33,188–194.

GESCHWIND, N. and GALABURDA, A. (1985). Cerebral lateralization. Biological mechanisms, associations and pathology. I, II and III. *Archives of Neurology*, 42, 428–459; 521–552; 634–654.

HARCHERIK, D. F., COHEN, D. J., ORT, S., PAUL, R., SHAYWITZ, B. A., VOLKMAR, F. R., ROTHMAN, S. L. G. and LECKMAN, J. F. (1985). Computed tomographic brain scanning in four neuropsychiatric disorders of childhood. *American Journal of Psychiatry*, 142, 731–734.

HASLAM, R.H.A., DALBY, J.T., JOHNS, R.D., and RADEMAKER, A.W. (1981). Cerebral asymmetry in developmental dyslexia. *Archives of Neurology*, 38, 679–682.

HAYNES, C. and NAIDOO, C. (1991). Children wih Specific Speech and Language Impairment. *Clinics in Developmental Medicine, 119*. London: Mac Keith Press.

HAY, D.A. (1985). *Essentials of Behaviour Genetics*. Melbourne: Blackwell Scientific.

HURST, J.A., BARAITSER, M., AUGER, E., GRAHAM, F. and NORELL, S. (1990). An extended family with a dominantly inherited speech disorder. *Developmental Medicine and Child Neurology*, 32, 352–355.

JERNIGAN, T., HESSELINK, J.R., SOWELL, E. and TALLAL, P. (1992). Cerebral morphology on MRI in language/learning impaired children. *Archives of Neurology* (in press).

KLEIN, J.O. (1986). Risk factors for otitis media in children. in J. Kavanagh (Ed.) *Otitis Media and Child Development*. Parkton, MD: York Press.

LOUS, J. (1990). Secretory otitis media and phonology when starting school. *Scandinavian Audiology*, 19, 215–222.

LOUS, J. and FIELLAU-NIKOLAJSEN, M. (1984). A five-year prospective case-control study of the influence of early otitis media with effusion on reading achievement. *International Journal of Pediatric Otorhinolaryngology*, 8, 19–30.

MOGFORD, K. (1988). Language development in twins. In D. Bishop and K. Mogford (Eds) *Language Development in Exceptional Circumstances*. Edinburgh: Churchill Livingstone.

MOGFORD, K. and BISHOP, D. (1988). Five questions about language acquisition considered in the light of exceptional circumstances. In D. Bishop and K. Mogford (Eds), *Language Development in Excepional Circumsances*. Edinburgh: Churchill Livingstone.

NEILS, J. and ARAM, D. (1986). Family history of children with developmental language disorders. *Perceptual and Motor Skills*, 63, 655–658.

NICHOLS, R. C. and BILBRO, W. C. (1966). The diagnosis of twin zygosity. *Acta Geneticae Medicae et Gemellologiae*, 16, 265–275.

PENNINGTON, B.F., SMITH, S.D., KIMBERLING, W.J., GREEN, P.A. and HAITH, M.M. (1987), Left-handedness and immune disorders in familial dyslexics. *Archives of Neurology*, 44, 634–639.

PLOMIN, R., DEFRIES, J.C. and MCCLEARN, G.E. (1990). *Behavioral Genetics*, 2nd edition. New York: W. H. Freeman.

RAVEN, J.C., COURT, J. H. and RAVEN, J. (1977). *Raven's Progressive Matrices*. London: H.K. Lewis.

RENFREW, C. (1980). *Word-finding Vocabulary Scale*. Oxford: C. E. Renfrew.

ROBERTS, J.E., SANYAL, M. A., BURCHINAL, M. R., COLLIER, A. M., RAMEY, C. T. and HENDERSON, F. w. (1986). Otitis media in early childhood and its relationships to later verbal and academic performance. *Pediatrics*, 78, 423–430.

ROBINSON, R.J. (1987). Introduction and overview. In: *Proceedings of the First International Symposium on Specific Speech and Language Disorders in Children*. London: AFASIC.

ROSENBERGER, P.B. and HIER, D. B. (1980). Cerebral asymmetry and verbal intellectual deficits. *Annals of Neurology*, 8, 300–304.

RUMSEY, J., DORWART, R., VERMESS, M., DENCKLA, M.B., KRUESI, M.J.P. and RAPOPORT, J. (1986). Magnetic resonance imaging of brain anatomy in severe developmental dyslexia. *Archives of Neurology*, 43, 1045–1046.

RUTTER, M., MACDONALD, H., LE COUTEUR, A., HARRINGTON, R., BOLTON, P. and BAILEY, A. (1990a). Genetic factors in child psychiatric disorders – II. Empirical findings. *Journal of Child Psychology and Psychiatry*, 31, 39–83.

RUTTER, M., BOLTON, P., HARRINGTON, R., LE COUTEUR, A., MACDONALD, H. and SIMONOFF, E. (1990b). Genetic factors in child psychiatric disorders – I. A review of research strategies. *Journal of Child Psychology and Psychiatry*, 31, 3–37.

SCHIFF-MYERS, N. (1988). Hearing children of deaf parents. In: D. Bishop and K. Mogford (Eds), *Language Development in Exceptional Circumstances*. Edinburgh: Churchill Livingstone.

SEMEL, E. M. and WIIG, E. H. (1980). *Clinical Evaluaion of Language Functions*. Columbus, OH: Merrill.

SHARE, D. L., CHALMERS, D., SILVA, P. A. and STEWART, I. A. (1986). Reading disability and middle ear disease. *Archives of Disease in Childhood*, 61, 400–410.

SILVA, P. A., CHALMERS, D. and STEWART, I. (1986). Some audiological, educational and behavioral characteristics of children with bilateral otitis media with effusion – a longitudinal study. *Journal of Learning Disabilities*, 19, 165–169.

TALLAL, P., ROSS, R. and CURTISS, S. (1989). Familial aggregation in specific language impairment. *Journal of Speech and Hearing Disorders*, 54, 167–173.

TEELE, D. W., KLEIN, J. O., ROSNER, B. A. and THE GREATER BOSTON OTITIS MEDIA STUDY GROUP (1984). Otitis media with effusion during the first three years of life and development of speech and language. *Pediatrics*, 74, 282–287.

TOMBLIN, J. B. (1989). Familial concentration of developmental language impairment. *Journal of Speech and Hearing Disorders*, 54, 287–295.

WADSWORTH, S. J., GILLIS, J. J., DEFRIES, J. C. and FULKER, D. W. (1989). Differential genetic aetiology of reading disability as a function of age. *Irish Journal of Psychology*, 10, 509–520.

WECHSLER, D. (1974). *Wechsler Intelligence Scale for Children – Revised*. New York: The Psychological Corporation.

# Chapter 2
# Qualitative differences in the conversational interactions of SLI children and their younger siblings

GRAEME D. HUTCHESON AND GINA CONTI-RAMSDEN*

## Introduction

It has been consistently demonstrated that adult interaction with children differs significantly from adult–adult interaction; in the study of Anglo-American language learning children (see Snow, Perlman and Nathan, 1987, for a review), in the study of adult–child interaction in different cultures (Brice Heath, 1983; Ochs, 1982; Schieffelin, 1979) and in the study of atypical language learners and their parents (see Conti-Ramsden, 1985, for a review). What these differences entail, on the other hand, has not always been clear. The special features of parent–child interaction are quite culturally specific (Snow, Perlman and Nathan, 1987), and some features are likely to have facilitative effects for language learning while others seem to offer no particular advantage to the task of cracking the linguistic code (Snow, 1989). The characteristics of the child, for example whether the child has a language problem or not, may also affect the nature of parent–child interaction (Horsborough, Cross and Ball, 1985; Conti-Ramsden, 1990). This latter argument is of particular interest to clinician-researchers interested in language impairment, as it has implications for assessment and remediation.

Previous research has focused on examining common features of adult–child interaction in different groups of atypical language learners (Horsborough, Cross and Ball, 1985), and on examining differences between specific language-impaired (SLI) parent–child dyads and normal control dyads (Cross, 1981; Conti-Ramsden and Friel-Patti, 1983; 1984; Cross, Nienhuys and Kirkman, 1985). Comparative research with

* This research is supported by a March of Dimes Research Foundation grant (no. 12-251) made to the second author.

normal control children has suggested that mothers of SLI children may initiate more interaction, in order to compensate for their children who tend to be less able to initiate conversation than normal control children of the same language stage (Conti-Ramsden and Friel-Patti, 1983; 1984). In addition, Cross and her colleagues (Cross, 1981; Cross, Nienhuys and Kirkman, 1985) compared SLI with normal language learners of the same stage. The prediction was that mothers of SLI children when interacting with their younger offspring would not differ from a normal control group, supporting the position that it was the SLI child's special influence which brought about the differences in maternal speech. The results were thought provoking. Cross and her colleagues found that well over half the reliable differences between the SLI versus control mothers disappeared when mothers of language-impaired children interacted with their younger, normal offspring.

However, since in the Cross studies mothers of SLI children were compared with normal controls outside the family, there was no way of examining within-family consistencies and discrepancies. The aim of the present investigation was to further this line of research by examining a natural but infrequently occurring situation where a family has both an SLI child and a normal younger sibling of the same language stage. This methodological approach, which involves comparing mothers' interactions with their SLI children to the same mothers' interactions with their non-language-impaired children affords us an opportunity to begin to tease out the relative effects of the mother and the child on the nature of the interaction. In the present study the focus was mainly on the children and the nature of their interaction with their mothers. By keeping the control group within the same family we were able to ask questions such as: what characteristics of the children's speech (SLI versus normal) change in interaction with the mother? And what characteristics of children's speech (SLI versus normal sibling) are constant?

## Method

Six families with an SLI child and a younger sibling at a comparable mean length of utterance (MLU) level took part in this investigation. The data on four of the families (Charles and Clay, Kate and Kyle, Rick and Rose, Sid and Susan) were obtained through the Child Language database* and the other two (Jack and Jim, Martin and Mathue) were

---

*These recordings were originally made as part of an investigation by Conti-Ramsden and Dykins (1991). Charles is referred to as Chuck in the database. Copies of the data and information on CHILDES can be obtained from Brian McWhinney, Department of Psychology, Carnegie Mellon University, Pittsburgh, PA, 15215, USA, and in the UK from the second author (Dr Conti-Ramsden) or from Dr Martyn Barrett, Department of Psychology, Royal Holloway and Bedford New College, University of London, Egham Hill, Egham, Surrey, TW20 0EX.

recruited specifically for this project. The names of the children (which have been changed), their ages and their MLU scores are all given in Table 2.1.

**Table 2.1** Children's ages and MLU values

| Name | Age | Age difference | MLU | MLU difference |
|------|-----|----------------|-----|----------------|
| Clay [a] | 6;4.26 | | 1.216 | |
| Charles | 2;10.21 | 3;6.5 | 1.385 | 0.169 |
| Jack [a] | 4;10.25 | | 1.389 | |
| Jim | 2;4.8 | 2;6.17 | 1.543 | 0.154 |
| Kate [a] | 4;9.18 | | 2.165 | |
| Kyle | 2;4.21 | 2;4.28 | 2.069 | 0.096 |
| Martin [a] | 3;8.19 | | 1.167 | |
| Mathue | 2;1.4 | 1;7.15 | 1.351 | 0.184 |
| Rick [a] | 6;9.19 | | 2.298 | |
| Rose | 3;2.15 | 3;7.4 | 2.333 | 0.035 |
| Sid [a] | 4;9.8 | | 1.525 | |
| Susan | 2;7.6 | 2;2.2 | 1.228 | 0.297 |

[a] Language-impaired child. All names have been changed.

The SLI children and their younger siblings have been matched closely on MLU and are all within 0.3 morphemes of one another . The age differences between the children range from 1 year 7.5 months for Martin and Mathue, to just over 3 years 7 months for Rick and Rose. The MLU value calculated here is based on that used by Brown (1973) with the modifications suggested by Miller (1981)*.

All children were videotaped in their homes, and in order to keep the mothers as unconcerned as possible about their own speech they were told that the research was primarily about child language development. The instructions given to the mothers was to 'play as you normally do'.

The recordings were transcribed onto a computer in accordance with the guidelines produced by the Codes for Human Analysis of Transcript, or CHAT (MacWhinney and Snow, 1985). The original recordings were transcribed using CHAT version 0.7 (Conti-Ramsden and Dykins, 1991) and were updated to CHAT 1.0 in line with the two new families by the first author (all transcriptions are to be donated to the CHILDES

---

*All direct imitations and repetitions were omitted, as were rhymes and repetitive naming and counting. The morpheme count for utterances containing multiple conjunctions was restricted to the first fully formed structure (e.g. For the utterance 'I like him and her and that and that and that...' only 'I like him and her' are counted).

data-base in the near future). The transcriptions were all of 10 minutes duration. For more detailed information on the specific procedures and equipment used refer to Conti-Ramsden and Dykins (1991).

## The Coding Scheme

The coding scheme used to divide the transcriptions into separate utterances was based around the following definition of conversations: 'Two or more turns linked together by a focus on a particular topic' (Conti-Ramsden and Friel-Patti, 1987). The codes added to the transcriptions designated the initial and final utterance of a conversation ($NEW and $END) as well as all those in between ($CON).

This analysis is primarily concerned with identifying conversational breakdown and any differences in interactional style between children. To do this, a definition of 'topic change' had to be decided upon that could pick up on any breakdowns but wasn't so stringent as to class any relatively minor shifts in topic as breakdowns, or too broad, to miss many of the more subtle breakdowns. The scheme used here utilises the idea of a 'theme' to define a conversation. As long as an interaction is following a particular theme and there are no indications of a breakdown then it is regarded as being a single conversation.

The major indicators of breakdown are time gaps (more than 5 seconds between consecutive utterances strongly indicates that a particular conversation has ended), changes in the focus of the conversation or in the item under discussion, and changes in the function of the utterance (for example, changing from questions to commands). However, these are only *indicators* of breakdown and all information is taken into account in deciding if a conversation is continuing. For example, the presence of an imitation or repetition is taken to indicate that the participants are at least communicating about the same items, and without strong indications to the contrary this is enough to classify the interaction as being a conversation. The following interaction is coded as being a single conversation on the grounds that although it is unclear what the child is talking about when he says 'got big' and 'got big one there', there is some evidence linking these to his and his mother's former utterances ('got big' can be regarded as being a partial imitation or repetition):

```
*CHI:    got no window.
%act:    turns around and looks at lego car MOT is making
%cod:    $NEW
*MOT:    it-'has got no window.
*MOT:    it-'is not a <very good car then> [>].
%cod:    $CON
```

```
*CHI:    <got big> [<].
*CHI:    got big.
%cod:    $CON
*MOT:    there-'is the window.
%act:    continues making the model
%cod:    $CON
 *CHI:   got big one there.
%cod:    $END
```

Embedded or overlapping conversations can occur when the theme of the conversations changes but there is no breakdown. In cases such as this the interaction is coded as a single conversation. All unclear utterances and non-verbal responses are coded as turns in a conversation if there is any indication that the conversation is continuing. Multiple utterances by a single person are coded as being a single conversational turn (see the above example).

The majority of conversations in the transcripts were easy to identify as they had a relatively clear theme and tended to be terminated by a clear breakdown or were terminated normally without a breakdown (e.g. an answer to a question). The area where the coding becomes more subjective and open to different interpretations between different coders was in defining the scope of the theme reliably. There were, however, very few disagreements in the coding, as evidenced by a point-by-point reliability score of over 90% for two independent researchers coding a complete transcript.

**Results and Discussion**

Table 2.2 shows the total number of conversations and the average number of turns in each conversation for all of the children. A breakdown showing the status of the utterances which make up the conversations is presented. The total number of conversations includes those which have not been completely transcribed (those conversations at the start or end of the transcript; a maximum of two in any transcript) and the mean length is obtained by calculating the total number of utterances involved divided by the total number of conversations. Also included is the number of utterances which initiated, continued, or ended conversations. It should be noted here that the code $NEW refers to those utterances which actually began a conversation and not those that attempted to initiate one. The $END code only indicates the number of utterances which were the last in a conversation and does not indicate who was responsible for terminating the conversations.

The average length of conversations of the children and their mothers does not discriminate between the SLI children and their younger siblings. Three of the SLI children (Clay, Jack, and Martin) engaged in longer conversations with their mothers than did their younger siblings, whilst the other three (Kate, Rick, and Sid) engaged in shorter conversations. Neither the age of the children nor their MLU scores predict the length of their conversations for the group as a whole ($r= -0.04$, $P>0.05$; $r= -0.49$, $P>0.05$), or for the SLI ($r= -0.05$, $P>0.05$; $r= -0.8$, $P>0.05$) and siblings ($r= -0.06$, $P>0.05$; $r= 0.29$, $P>0.05$) separately.

**Table 2.2** Breakdown of conversations

| Name | No. Convs | Mean Length | CHI $NEW | MOT $NEW | CHI $CON | MOT $CON | CHI $END | MOT $END |
|------|------|------|------|------|------|------|------|------|
| Clay* | 26 | 5.92 | 3 | 23 | 57 | 45 | 10 | 16 |
| Charles | 38 | 4.05 | 18 | 20 | 45 | 33 | 7 | 31 |
| Jack* | 40 | 4.98 | 9 | 30 | 66 | 54 | 15 | 25 |
| Jim | 41 | 4.37 | 6 | 35 | 48 | 49 | 34 | 7 |
| Kate* | 46 | 3.76 | 17 | 29 | 47 | 34 | 16 | 30 |
| Kyle | 40 | 4.4 | 13 | 27 | 56 | 41 | 12 | 27 |
| Martin* | 30 | 5.3 | 1 | 29 | 62 | 38 | 5 | 24 |
| Mathue | 27 | 5.0 | 11 | 16 | 44 | 37 | 8 | 19 |
| Rick* | 34 | 3.65 | 10 | 24 | 32 | 24 | 16 | 18 |
| Rose | 28 | 4.96 | 8 | 19 | 44 | 40 | 15 | 13 |
| Sid* | 25 | 3.6 | 9 | 16 | 24 | 17 | 9 | 15 |
| Susan | 29 | 4.55 | 10 | 19 | 43 | 31 | 7 | 22 |

* Learning-impaired child.

Average length of conversation did not predict which children were impaired, their age, or their MLU level. It can be seen in Table 2.2 that there were indications of differences between the conversations that the SLI children and their siblings have with their mothers. The most noticeable difference between an SLI child and younger sibling was in the number of conversations which they initiated. Martin and Clay have both initiated far fewer conversations than their younger siblings; the other pairs, however, do not show any noticeable differences in the number of initiations that they made. The following discussion will concentrate on this particular difference between the two pairs Martin and Mathue, and Clay and Charles.

**Martin and Mathue**

These two children show the smallest difference in ages (19.5 months) when matched on MLU and have similar average conversation lengths (5.3 and 5.0 turns). The major apparent difference between the two children is in the number of conversations that they initiated; Martin (the SLI child) initiated 3.3% of all his conversations compared with Mathue's 40.7%. Nevertheless it is important to note that the volume of conversation is similar for both children with Martin using 74 utterances overall and engaging in 30 conversations compared with Mathue who uses 76 utterances overall and engages in 27 conversations.

The differences between the two children's results could be due to two main factors, or a combination of them. First, Martin might not be providing many opportunities for a conversation to be initiated and secondly, assuming that there *are* opportunities, his mother might not be picking up on them. To try and ascertain which of these explanations was more likely a simple analysis was carried out which involved categorising all of the children's utterances into one of two groups. Group 1 contained replies to direct questions, direct imitations, and 'noises' (e.g. 'vroom vroom') which do not appear to attempt to elicit an interaction. Group 2 contained any spontaneous utterance which could have initiated a conversation (no intent on the part of the child is needed), which included attention getters ('Mum', 'Oy'), unprompted naming of items, comments, questions and commands. The results of this analysis are given in Table 2.3.

**Table 2.3** Analysis of all utterances

|         | Group 1      | Group 2      |
|---------|--------------|--------------|
| Martin  | 70 (94.6%)   | 4 (5.4%)     |
| Mathue  | 53 (69.7%)   | 23 (30.3%)   |

We can see from Table 2.3 that the distribution of utterances between the two groups differed markedly. Martin's Group 2 utterances contained two examples of the word 'there' as he fixed pieces into a puzzle, one instance of spontaneous naming ('brick'), and an unintelligible utterance which appeared to be an attempt to get his mother's attention and initiated the conversation shown below:

```
*CHI:    xxx.
%act:    holds up piece of toy
%cod:    $NEW
*MOT:    that-'s a wall # is-'nt it?
%cod:    $CON
*CHI:    yeah.
%cod:    $CON
```

Mathue, on the other hand, had many more utterances in Group 2 (30.3%) and these resulted in the initiation of 11 conversations during the recording. The spontaneous utterances that Mathue used most were attention getters such as 'Mummy', naming and describing items (e.g. 'red one' when picking up a red counter), and some direct commands ('look!' and 'don't!'). Mathue also showed four examples of repeating spontaneous utterances when they weren't replied to. In the following example Mathue's mother is handing him some toys from a box and does not pick up on his initial comment about one of the toys being broken:

```
*MOT:   have another train.
%act:   hands Mathue another train
*CHI:   come off.
%act:   toy has fallen apart
*MOT:   another train.
*CHI:   come off.
%cod:   $NEW
*MOT:   oh # has it come off?
%cod:   $CON
```

As can be seen, Mathue (the younger sibling) repeats himself until he gets his mother to attend to and participate in his conversation.

## Clay and Charles

Clay and Charles show a similar pattern to Martin and Mathue in that there is a relatively large difference in the number of conversations they initiate (3 and 18 respectively). The age difference between Clay and Charles is, however, greater than for Martin and Mathue. Clay's impairment would appear to be more severe (he is 42.5 months older). Conversations were initiated by Clay (the SLI child) 11.5% of the time whilst Charles initiated 47.4% of his conversations. The results of an analysis of all utterances made by Clay and Charles in the same way as was done for Martin and Mathue can be seen in Table 2.4.

**Table 2.4** Analysis of all utterances

|         | Group 1   | Group 2  |
|---------|-----------|----------|
| Clay    | 68        | 7        |
|         | (90.7%)   | (9.3%)   |
| Charles | 48        | 32       |
|         | (60.0%)   | (40.0%)  |

We can see from Table 2.4 that both children make a similar number of utterances (80 and 75) and the distribution of utterances between the two groups is similar to that seen for Martin and Mathue. Clay makes only seven spontaneous utterances, two of which are of unclear status, two are spontaneous naming, two are comments when picking up puzzle pieces ('there'), and one is a call for attention ('Mum'). Charles gives many more opportunities for conversations to start and these include numerous examples of spontaneous naming, attention getters, and comments ('um off # lid' [taking lid off saucepan], and 'Ruth got it' [wants chair that Ruth is sitting on]). Charles also repeats some utterances when they were not originally met with a reply. For example:

| | |
|---|---|
| *CHI: | um Clay-'s. |
| %act: | reaching for toy in MOT's hand |
| *MOT: | there. |
| %act: | puts toy on floor |
| *CHI: | Clay-'s. |
| *CHI: | Clay-'s. |
| %act: | points to truck on the floor |
| *MOT: | yeah. |
| *MOT: | is that Clay-'s? |
| *CHI: | yeah. |

This 'strategy' of the younger sibling involving repetition until attention and engagement by the mother in the conversation is obtained seems to work for the dyad.

**General Discussion**

The two pairs investigated have shown the same basic patterns in their conversational behaviour and, despite the preliminary nature of these results, some discussion is warranted. Although the SLI children were compared with a younger sibling at a similar stage of development (as measured by MLU) there were marked differences in what the children said. The analysis in Tables 2.3 and 2.4 were quite crude, with the two groups defined to show any possible initiations, whether they were intended as such or not. The results showed that this distinction was sufficient to distinguish between the children, as nearly all of the SLI children's speech was answers to direct questions or direct imitations, which were capable of keeping conversations going, but which did not result in many initiations. This is much like Conti-Ramsden and Friel-Patti's (1983) finding that SLI children appear to be more passive.

Nevertheless, this difference between some of the language-impaired children and their younger siblings is unlikely to apply to all the pairs in the study, as many show no differences in the number of initiations. Recent research on individual differences in the conversations of mothers and their SLI and younger offspring (Conti-Ramsden and Dykins, 1991) suggests that SLI children can not be treated as a group. They found that despite significant group results, individual styles of interaction were marked and entirely different for different families. We have demonstrated that, for at least two of the pairs in this study, there is a qualitative difference between the children's interactions with their mother that is not indicated by MLU value or the average size of conversations. We have also argued that a more in-depth, detailed analysis of the structure and the content of SLI children's conversations reveals important individual differences and provides a better picture of what is at stake in parent–child interaction.

## References

BRICE HEATH, S. (1983).*Ways with words*. Cambridge: Cambridge University Press.

BROWN, R. (1973). *A First Language*. Cambridge, MA: Harvard University Press.

CONTI-RAMSDEN, G. (1985). Mothers in dialogue with language-impaired children. *Topics in Language Disorders*, **5**, 58–68.

CONTI-RAMSDEN, G. (1990). Recasts and other contingent replies to language-impaired children. *Journal of Speech and Hearing Disorders*, **55**, 262–274.

CONTI-RAMSDEN, G. and DYKINS, J. (1991). Mother-child interaction with language-impaired children and their siblings. *British Journal of Disorders of Communication*, **26**, 337–354

CONTI-RAMSDEN, G. and FRIEL-PATTI, S. (1983). Mothers' discourse adjustments to language-impaired and non-language-impaired children. *Journal of Speech and Hearing Disorders*, **48**, 360–367.

CONTI-RAMSDEN, G. and FRIEL-PATTI, S. (1984). Mother–child dialogues: A comparison of normal and language-impaired children. *Journal of Communication Disorders*, **17**, 19–35.

CONTI-RAMSDEN, G. and FRIEL-PATTI, S. (1987). Situational variability in mother–child conversations. In: Nelson, K.E. and van Kleeck, A. (Eds), *Children's Language*, Vol 6. Hillsdale, NJ: Lawrence Erlbaum Associates.

CROSS, T.G. (1981). The linguistic experience of slow learners. In:Nesdale, A.R., Pratt, C., Grieve, R., Field, J., Illingworth, D. and Hogben, J. (Eds), *Advances in Child Development: Theory and Research* (pp. 110–121). Proceedings of the First National Conference on Child Development, University of Western Australia, Nedlands, Australia.

CROSS, T.G., NIENHUYS, T. G. and KIRKMAN, M. (1985). Parent–child interaction with receptively disabled children: some determinants of Maternal Speech Style. In: Nelson, K. (Ed.), *Children's Language*, Vol 5 (pp.247–289). New York: Gardner Press.

HORSBOROUGH, K., CROSS, T. and BALL, J. (1985). Conversational interaction between mothers and their autistic dysphasic and normal children. In: Cross, T.G. and Riach, L.M. (Eds), *Issues and Research in Child Development* (pp. 470–476). Proceedings of the Second National Child Development Conference, The Institute of Early Childhood Development, Melbourne College of Advanced Education, Victoria, Australia.

MACWHINNEY, B. and SNOW, C.E. (1985). The Child Language Data Exchange System. *Journal of Child Language*, **12**, 271–295.

MILLER, J.F. (1981). *Assessing Language Production in Children: Experimental Procedures*. University Park Press, Baltimore.

OCHS, E. (1982). Talking to children in Western Samoa. *Language in Society*, **11**, 77–104.

SCHIEFFELIN, B. B. (1979). Getting it together: An ethnographic approach to the study of the development of communicative competence. In Ochs, E. and Schiefflin, B.B. (Eds), *Developmental Pragmatics*. New York: Academic Press.

SNOW, C. E. (1989). Understanding social interaction and language acquisition; sentences are not enough. In: Bornstein, M. H. and Bruner, J. S. (Eds), *Interaction in Human Development* (pp.83–103), Hillsdale, NJ: Lawrence Erlbaum Associates.

SNOW, C.E., PERLMAN, R. and NATHAN, D. (1987). Why routines are different: Towards a multiple factors model of relation between input and language acquisition. In: Nelson, K. and van Kleeck, A. (Eds), *Children's Language*, Vol 6. Hillsdale, NJ: Lawrence Erlbaum Associates.

# Chapter 3
# The relationship between deprivation, physical growth and the impaired development of language

DAVID SKUSE

Physical growth and the development of language in childhood are both critically dependent on the provision of appropriate attention and stimulation by a caretaker. In general terms, we would anticipate that there is a minimal necessary degree of exposure to appropriate nurturance in these respects in order to promote a rate of growth and an acquisition of linguistic skills that is well within the range of normal for any given society. Over the past 50 years or so quite a substantial literature has grown up on the subject of the effects of so-called deprivation, including neglect and abuse both by parents and within institutions, upon child development. Yet there is a substantial dichotomy in what has been written between those who have studied the children's physical development – usually paediatricians, writing for medical journals, and those who have studied the children's psychological development, especially language – a topic that has attracted the attention of psychologists and social scientists. Rarely has it been noticed that those very children whose growth is impaired tend also to have delayed language. Conversely, children with impaired cognitive skills secondary to an impoverished upbringing do seem to be rather small for their age. It is my intention first to draw together these diverse strands and show that, were we to look for it more assiduously, the association between impaired physical growth and language skills would be found more often and secondly to demonstrate that there is good evidence that removal of affected children from their depriving circumstances into a more advantageous situation can result in an accelerated rate of development of both growth and language, if we care to measure change longitudinally. Thirdly, I will discuss what features of that advantaged environment would be sufficient and necessary to promote what we might call 'catch-up growth' in these attributes. Fourthly, I will comment on the evidence for the existence of so-called sensitive periods for physical growth and language skills, deprivation during which can lead to long-lasting, possibly permanent, detrimental consequences.

Let us start by considering the effects upon development of an upbringing in conditions of near total lack of stimulation and nurture. There are some marvellous historical accounts, based on the fact that over many centuries, and indeed millennia, man has considered that a careful analysis of the sequelae of extreme deprivation of human contact in early childhood might reveal valuable insights into how normal language develops. To this end children have occasionally been deliberately raised in conditions of extreme isolation.

Such experiments were said to have been attempted by the Holy Roman Emperor, Frederick II, and King James IV of Scotland. Unfortunately, not only did the children in these studies fail to develop comprehensible speech but those in Frederick II's experiment, which was designed to see whether children to whom no one had spoken would first speak Hebrew, Greek, Latin, Arabic or the language of their parents, all died. This is said (Ross and McLaughlin, 1949) to have been attributable to the fact that 'they had been cut off from human speech "because they could not live without the petting and the joyful faces and loving words of their foster mothers, or without those swaddling songs" which a woman sings to put a child to sleep, without which "it sleeps badly and has no rest".' I would lay a heavy bet that those children not only failed to develop language, but that they failed to thrive physically as well.

There are, in addition, a number of reports within our own times concerning individual children who spent their early years in conditions of extreme impoverishment and deprivation as a result of deliberate actions by nefarious, ignorant or incompetent caregivers (Skuse, 1989a; b).

One such case would do well for illustrative purposes; it is known to be a classic study of how cognitive development may be seriously impaired by early deprivation yet later recover, apparently fully, on cessation of that deprivation and the restoration of the affected children to a stimulating and loving environment. What is not so well known is that exactly equivalent observations could be made of the children's growth (Koluchova, 1979). Jarmila Koluchova initially reported in 1972 (Koluchova, 1972; 1976) the case records of monozygotic male twins, who were born on 4 September 1960. Their mother had died shortly after giving birth and for 11 months they lived in a children's home. They then spent 6 months with a maternal aunt but were subsequently taken to live with their father and stepmother. For 5 years, until their discovery at the age of 7, the twins lived under most abnormal conditions, in a quiet street of family houses in Czechoslovakia. Because of the actions of their stepmother, who had her own children whom she actively preferred, the boys grew up in almost *total* isolation, never being allowed out of the house but living in a small unheated closet. They were often locked up for long periods in the summer, sleeping on the floor on a plastic sheet, and they were cruelly chastised. When discovered at the age of 7 they could barely walk and suffered from acute rickets. They showed reactions of surprise and horror to objects and activities normally very familiar to children of that age, such as moving mechanical toys, a television set or traffic in the street. Their spontaneous speech was very poor, as was their play.

After discovery and removal the boys were placed at first in hospital, where they remained for a few weeks before going to a small children's home. Their mental age was initially around the 3 year level, whereas their chronological age was 7;3 years. After approximately 18 months in the children's home they were placed in a foster family with whom they remained until adulthood. Tremendous gains in cognitive attainments were made within a few months of their rescue and a further significant increase in the rate of improvement occurred on transfer to the foster home. The long-term outcome was excellent and the boys developed above average linguistic skills as well as making good socioemotional adjustment to adolescence (Figures 3.1 and 3.2). What is evident from these trajectories of recovery in growth in terms of both height and IQ is how closely the two match each other, not only in terms of the rate of recovery but also in terms of the rate of change within each individual, so that the tempo of recovery is rather more rapid for Paul than it was for John.

This association between severe neglect and impaired physical and mental development has been seen in other circumstances, where the degree of environmental adversity was by no means as severe as it had been for the twins studied by Koluchova. There has for some time been a recognition that speech and language ability will be impaired among children who have been abused and neglected by their caretakers. In some cases there is coincident impairment of physical growth but this is rarely recognised. For example, it is notable that in a recent major textbook on child maltreatment (Ciccietti and Carlson, 1989) the index contains several references to the deleterious effects of abuse and neglect upon the development of language but no entry at all on 'growth', although a couple of entries are found for 'failure to thrive'.

Emotional abuse and neglect of children may take many forms, from lack of care for their physical needs, through a failure to provide consistent love and nurture, to overt hostility and rejection. Deleterious effects upon developing children are correspondingly diverse and tend to vary

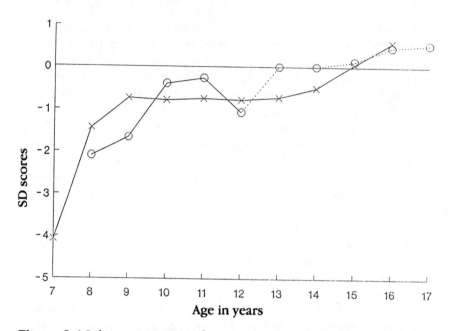

**Figure 3.1** John: trajectories of recovery in terms of verbal skills and linear growth, measured in standard deviation scores. x, Height; —— verbal IQ; - - - full scale IQ.

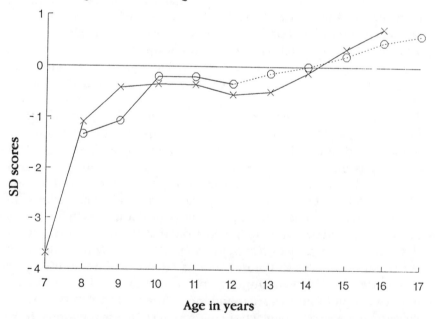

**Figure 3.2** Paul: trajectories of recovery in terms of verbal skills and linear growth, measured in standard deviation scores. x, Height; —— verbal IQ; - - - full scale IQ.

with age. In infancy, neglect is likely to be associated with developmental delays, of which delay in language development will be a predominant symptom. Preschool children may additionally present with disorders of social and emotional adjustment. 'Neglect' comprises both a lack of physical caretaking and supervision, and a failure to engage the developmental needs of the child in terms of cognitive stimulation. It is often associated with emotional abuse, by which I mean the habitual verbal harassment of a child by disparagement, criticism, threat and ridicule – and the inversion of love; by verbal and non-verbal means, rejection and withdrawal are substituted (Skuse, 1989a). Although direct observations of parenting may raise suspicions about the presence of emotional abuse and neglect, the diagnosis is usually suggested by its consequences for the child; important features that should be readily observable include impaired growth, especially short stature, and exceptionally poor language skills.

During infancy the neglect of physical and emotional nurture is likely to be manifest in those aspects of physical development that demand the closest attention from caregivers. Babies are dependent creatures; they need to be fed regularly, to be kept in a reasonably dry and warm environment, and to have their bowel and bladder functions taken care of. If they arc not fed adequately they will fail to thrive. Failure to thrive is usually defined as an exceptionally poor rate of growth in which weight (and often length) become increasingly divergent from normal age standardised values (Skuse, 1985). The physical consequences of persistent neglect through the preschool period often include poor growth, not only in terms of height and weight but also in head circumference. When there has been serious and persistent neglect, social and psychomotor skills are also likely to be affected. Normal infants are innately sociable but a severely neglected infant will not have learned the joy of reciprocal smiling and laughter, and may not attempt to elicit attention.

The development of communication between children, even those who cannot talk, and their caregivers is a subtle process with its own set of shared expectations and rules of operation. Persistent neglect and abuse will prevent the establishment of a 'mutual faith in a shared world'. Retardation in development of receptive and expressive language is very likely to result, possibly exacerbated by recurrent inadequately treated middle-ear infections and partial deafness. When emotional abuse has been severe a child may become virtually mute.

There is growing evidence that psychological, rather than physical, maltreatment could be the core reason for detriment to developmental outcomes in abused and neglected children (Claussen and Crittenden, 1991). It could also be the crucial factor responsible for impaired growth (Skuse, 1989b).

The association between reversible failure of both statural and mental growth with child abuse was first recognised at the Johns Hopkins Hospital by Money and his colleagues (Money, Annecillo and Kelley, 1983). The syndrome they described, which they termed 'abuse dwarfism', has no pathonomic signs or symptoms; it is the combination of current and historical features that is characteristic. Some aspects, such as certain behavioural characteristics, are rather distinctive. There may be no physical signs of abuse other than the short stature. The underlying aetiology is probably always dysfunctional secretion of growth hormone, and this diagnosis can be confirmed by appropriate laboratory testing (Stanhope et al., 1988; Skuse, 1989a).

Money and his colleagues observed that when children with the condition were rescued from their abusing families the rate of statural growth accelerated, and they went through a period of rapid 'catch-up growth'. The meaning of that term is as follows. In favourable environmental conditions the trajectory of growth in height of children is so constant that it may be represented by a relatively simple mathematical curve (Preece and Baines, 1978). Should adverse circumstance supervene, such as a severe and persistent illness, the rate of growth starts temporarily to slow down. After rectification of the disorder a phase of more rapid or accelerated growth is observed, which persists until the child's height and/or weight is back on the pre-existing trajectory (Tanner, 1986) (Figure 3.3). Some children will catch up very quickly, others may take relatively longer, yet eventually most end up back on the predicted trajectory. In general, the more severe the growth-retarding influence, the longer it acts, and the earlier in life it occurs, the worse the ultimate outcome. The fascinating characteristic of this phenomenon is

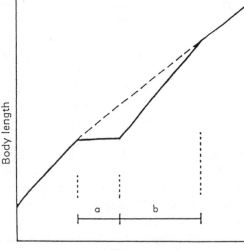

**Figure 3.3** 'Catch-up growth'. a, period of growth retardation; b, period of catch-up.

that, somehow, the growth-retarded child recognises that it is small. But it also recognises when it is restored to normal size – since, when approaching the normal curve, the rate of growth slows down and settles back onto it, no overshoot occurring in stature. The apparent reason for 'catch-up growth' in these formerly abused children seems to be that both the deficient secretion of growth hormone and the abnormally low rate of linear growth rapidly resolve when the child is removed from the abusive environment (Stanhope et al., 1988).

Money and colleagues found that the rate of change in mental growth seemed to run parallel to that of physical development, and was reflected in a progressive increase in intelligence, as measured by a standardised IQ test. They hypothesised that progressive catch-up growth in intelligence would be reflected in a positive correlation between the amount of IQ increase and the amount of time spent free of abuse after having been rescued (Figure 3.4). Of course, the children were rescued at various ages, and they had various degrees of developmental retardation at that time. In order to take account of the variability in age, baseline IQ and duration between rescue and the follow-up examination, a multiple regression analysis was undertaken. This showed that just three variables accounted for 60% of the variance in the elevation of IQ. Time after rescue accounted for most of the variance, as compared with baseline IQ

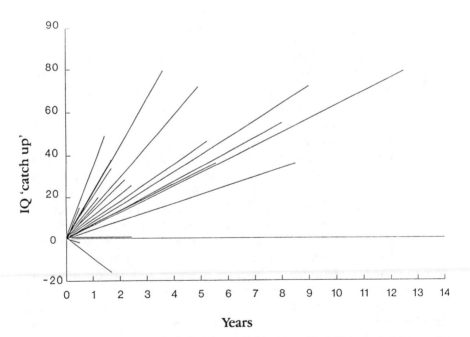

**Figures 3.4** Baseline to follow-up change in IQ among children who were rescued from abusing homes (Money, Annecillo and Kelley, 1983).

level, and baseline age acted as a moderator variable. The moderating role of age means that the younger the age at the time of rescue, the greater the amount of IQ elevation during a comparable period of time after rescue. Overall, the analysis showed that post-rescue growth of IQ was not sudden but was progressive over time. There was also evidence that the younger the age at rescue the greater the gains in IQ; children who were less than 5 years of age at rescue (*n*=7) gained an average of 33 points (± 24) during a follow-up period of 3;11 years, whereas those older than 5 years (*n*=7) gained in average only 16 points (± 7) during a follow-up period of 4;1 years. This was despite the fact that baseline IQs of the younger sample were slightly higher (71± 21) than those of the older sample (63± 15). Money does not specifically discuss language skills, but does present a case study of one girl who was rescued at the age of 3;8 years and whose verbal IQ was, on the Wechsler scales (Wechsler, 1976) 74 at 6;8 years. Yet it had risen to 126 at age 13;11 years, and her full-scale IQ had increased from 36 at discovery (Stanford-Binet form L-M; Terman and Merrill, 1960) to 120 at the time of the later follow up. Clearly gains of the magnitude made by the Koluchova twins are not particularly uncommon.

Regrettably, Money and co-workers do not discuss the degree of catch-up growth that is likely to have accompanied this improved intellectual performance. However, they state 'Catch-up statural growth (is a) most central criterion for the establishment of the diagnosis'.

The subject of the association between growth retardation, intellectual performance and catch-up growth in a large sample of abused and neglected children has also been well documented by Leonard Taitz and colleagues at the Children's Hospital in Sheffield (King and Taitz, 1985; Taitz and King, 1988a, b). They report a consecutive series of 260 children referred over the period between 1975 and 1986, with a variety of abuses. A retrospective analysis of case records revealed that 26% showed impairment of growth in terms of weight or height, and 14% had 'severely restricted' linear growth, being more than two standard deviatons below the population mean (Tanner, Whitehouse and Takaishi, 1966). Out of 11 such children placed in foster homes, 10 subsequently demonstrated significant catch-up growth. A typical picture of alterations in the rate of linear growth that can be observed according to changes in domicile is given by the following account of a child whose development I have followed for over a decade (Figure 3.5). It concerns a girl whose growth was severely impaired because of abuse and neglect in the first few years of life. Her mother was eventually referred for an expert opinion to the growth clinic at Great Ormond Street Hospital at which time the child was 4 years of age. When told by the paediatrician whom she consulted (it happened to be Professor Jim Tanner) that the answer to the child's growth problem was to give her daughter greater love and

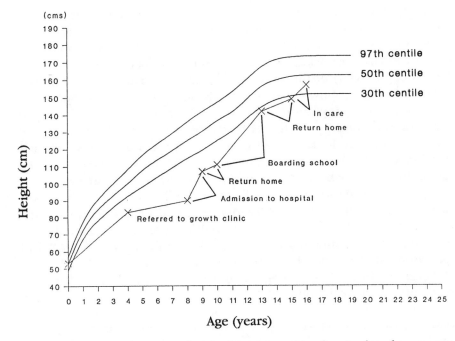

**Figure 3.5** Growth curve of girl with 'abuse dwarfism' related to events in her life. Her mother's height was 158 cm (25th centile) and her father's 178 cm (50th centile).

nutrition, the mother refused to come back. She was not seen again until some years later when the child was admitted to hospital, now aged 9 years, for investigation of possible growth hormone deficiency. That was when I first became involved. After the hormonal investigation failed to reveal any significant abnormality I arranged for her admission for 2 months to an inpatient unit for children with emotional and behavioural problems. It can be seen from Figure 3.5 that there was a relatively rapid increase in height (about 5 cm) in hospital, without any medication. Unfortunately, but predictably, the rate of growth slowed again once she returned home. She was subsequently admitted to a boarding school for 3 years, when she grew in term times only. Then her family moved away from the area and we lost touch with her until eventually, when she was 15 years of age, she ran away from home and asked to be taken into care. Finally, living away from her abusive home environment, her height eventually reached the 25th centile. That child had initially been in a school for children with moderate learning difficulties whilst living at home, but subsequently had a mainstream education. I met her again very recently and was delighted to find she is a warm, self-confident young woman who is planning to go into further education with the aim of becoming a community worker with mentally handicapped children.

The findings of Taitz et al. on the association between delays in mental development, including speech and language, and growth are of particular interest although the nature of the study and patient population means that their precision of measurement fell rather short of the ideal. A total of 87 (34%) of the series of 260 abused or neglected children were said to have shown evidence of developmental or language delay, or both. But the proportion within that subset of children with growth problems was considerably higher than those who did not have impaired growth. For example, among all those with growth problems 54% had developmental delays, whereas among those who had suffered non-accidental injury but whose growth was not impaired the figure was 22%. Compared with remaining cases in the series the children with growth problems had, on average, a 3.29-fold increased risk of developmental delay (95% confidence intervals 1.79 – 6.05). Emotional deprivation was especially closely linked with developmental delay, with a 13.8-fold increased risk (95% confidence intervals 7.1 – 27.1).

Severe degrees of neglect are of course not confined to families, and many of the early classical studies on the effects of severely understimulating environments upon child development were studies of children raised in institutional care. Once again, the detrimental effects of such an upbringing on mental development are well known, but what has not been emphasised or even discussed in commentaries on these pioneering studies is that there were parallel and equally severe deficits in the children's physical development.

For example, take René Spitz's original paper on 'Hospitalism', published in 1945 (Spitz, 1945a). He describes the severely impaired development of infants brought up in a foundling home somewhere in Latin America – the exact location of which has incidentally never been made explicit. The physical conditions of the home were described as follows: the children were placed, after spending the first 3 months in a newborn's ward, in individual cubicles that were enclosed by glass on three sides and open at the end. However, the glass panes did not begin until about 18" above the side rails of the cot. There they spent the first 15–18 months of their lives. Half were located in a dimly lit part of the ward, half in a well-lit section. 'Excellent food' is said to have been prepared, and all the children were breast fed in the first 3 months 'as a matter of principle'. Yet despite adequate physical care the children's environment was exceedingly monotonous and lacking in stimulation. No toys were available, the view from the cots was of a 'bleak and deserted' corridor. Bed sheets were routinely hung over the foot and side railings of the cots so that the children were effectively screened off from the world around them, and the only object visible was the ceiling. The babies lay supine for months, and eventually a hollow was worn into the mattresses so that they could not turn in any direction. The staff comprised one head and five assistant nurses for a total of 45 babies; no especial attempt was made to stimulate the children and Spitz observed 'the babies of the foundling home ...lack all human contact for most of the day'. In fact, human contact was limited to feeding times.

Although their developmental quotients were reported to be well above average in the first few months of life, by the end of the first year these had fallen to far below the normal range. Spitz recounts 'in the ward of the children ranging from 18 months to 2 years only 2 of the 26 surviving children spoke a couple of words. The same two are able to walk. A third child is beginning to walk. Hardly any of these can eat alone. Cleanliness habits have not been acquired and all are incontinent'. He remarks 'how much this deterioration could have been arrested if the children were taken out of the institution at the end of the first year is an open question. The fact that they remain in foundling homes probably furthers this progressive process. By the end of the second year the developmental quotient sinks to 45, which corresponds to a mental age of approximately 10 months, and would qualify these children as imbeciles' (Spitz, 1945a).

In a further paper (Spitz, 1945b) data are given on follow-up measures over a further 2 years and the following information is given on their speech development: virtually no child could speak more than 3–5 words (see Table 3.1). On this occasion physical measurements were made of weight, height and head circumference. The 21 remaining subjects (others had been adopted or given back to their families) were aged between 2 years and 4;1 years). 'Of all these children only 3 fall into the weight range of a normal *two year old* child, and only 2 have attained a length of a normal child of that age. All others fall below the normal two-year level – in one case as much as 45% in weight and 5" in length. In

**Table 3.1** Hospitalism: A follow-up report

| Speech Development | No. of Children |
| --- | --- |
| Cannot talk at all | 6 |
| Vocabulary: 2 words | 5 |
| Vocabulary: 3–5 words | 8 |
| Vocabulary: 12 words | 1 |
| Uses sentences | 1 |
| Total | 21 |
| Age range (years) | |
| 2;4–2;8 | 12 |
| 2;8–3;2 | 4 |
| 3;4–4;1 | 5 |

From Spitz, 1945b.

other words, the physical picture of these children impresses the casual observer as that of children half their age.'

Although Spitz's observations are now merely of historical interest in relation to the deprivation suffered by children in institutions in most parts of the developed world, this is by no means the case in Eastern Europe and the Soviet Union. Recently published harrowing pictures of infants and young children in Rumanian orphanages serve to remind us that severe impairments in mental and physical maturation can still be found, and are likely to result from similar aetiologies. This is a matter that has not only attracted the attention of the Western press, but is of great concern to researchers in those countries still possessing crèches and children's homes of this nature (Zdanska-Brincken et al., 1983; Chernova, 1990).

Studies have been presented to show that, in conditions of extreme deprivation, abuse and neglect, and poor quality institutional care, young children are often retarded in their physical development and, especially, in their acquisition of language. Is it likely that such an association would only be observed when a child's upbringing has been *so* neglectful or abusive that those circumstances would be encountered rarely, if at all, in homes that offer an 'average expectable environment'?

Some light is shed on this matter by a study conducted in a socially disadvantaged health district in South London (Dowdney et al., 1987; Heptinstall et al., 1987). We aimed to analyse prospective data on the growth trajectories of some 2000 children born in a single calendar year, with a view to selecting those with the most retarded height and weight at the age of 4 years. Cases were matched to a comparison group of children who were growing normally. Selection criteria stipulated that subjects should be full-term singleton births (gestation >38 weeks), without organic disease or disorder. Because it was wished to reduce heterogeneity on variables that were not under investigation the study was restricted to the 1200 Caucasian infants that had been born in 1980, the index year, of whom just over 70% were full-term. When they were seen, within a few weeks of their fourth birthdays, the case subjects were on average two standard deviations below the population mean for their height and weight, and were equivalently stunted when their parents' height was taken into account.

All subjects and their families received a comprehensive assessment – over 20 hours of investigations into their psychological and family functioning were made by interviewers and observers who were blind to the case status of the children. When we came to examine the developmental quotients of this group of proportionately small children we found a very worrying picture. On the McCarthy Scales of Children's Abilities they scored on average nearly 20 points below the comparison group (McCarthey, 1972). Nearly one-third scored below 70 and may for practical purposes be regarded as mild to moderately mentally handicapped. Only two children scored over 100 and the remainder were fairly evenly spread between scores of 50 to 100 so there was *no* excess of children with very low IQs pulling down the mean. The McCarthy Scales have recently been restandardised in the UK (Lynch et al., 1982) and if we recompute the children's full-scale scores in terms of standard deviations from the revised means we find that the cases scored, on average, nearly two standard deviations below the mean. Expressing their height for age in standard deviation scores as well we come up with an almost identical figure. However, despite the close similarity in the means, a regression analysis shows the correlation between their physical and mental development to be non-significant. The equivalent figures are not quite so striking among the comparison subjects.

We followed the children through their first years at school, and have some information about their outcome at 6 years of age. By that time nearly one-quarter of the cases were considered to be suffering from severe developmental delay and several had already undergone educational special needs assessments. A similar proportion had delayed development of speech, often in association with a clinically significant articulation difficulty, and had required speech therapy.

These findings of an association between impaired growth and developmental delays within a socioeconomically disadvantaged birth cohort are reflected in the reports of the Newcastle upon Tyne '1000 family' study, another longitudinal birth cohort survey, that commenced in 1947 (Kolvin et al., 1990). From the findings of that survey the authors conclude that there was an association between social deprivation and reduced height and weight that was due to postnatal growth. In addition, they present data to show that 'speech defects' were present in over 30% of their 'deprived' and 'multiply deprived' population, in comparison with just 18% in the 'non-deprived sample'.

We also obtained data on that proportion of our original birth cohort who had come to the attention of social services for neglect or abuse over the decade following their birth (Skuse, Wolke and Reilly, 1990). From these data we would be able to see whether the increased risk of developmental delay and speech and language difficulties in our group of growth-impaired children could be accounted for by the fact that they were more likely to have come from exceptionally disordered home circumstances, and hence would fall into the same category of children who were described by Taitz and his colleagues (Taitz and King, 1988a, b). We found that there was indeed an increased likelihood of children who persistently failed to thrive coming to the attention of social services, and their names being entered on a child protection register. The order of risk was increased about six times.

In some cases this professional concern was engendered by the growth disorder itself. But overall, it was only a minority – about 1 in 12 of such infants, who were known to have been seriously abused or neglected.

Returning to the questions posed at the outset of this chapter: first, if we look for it, we *do* seem to find an association between impaired physical growth and delayed or disordered speech and language skills in many children who are growing up in conditions of social deprivation. The association is most strong, and the degree of impairment most extreme, where the environment of upbringing is not only extremely impoverished – in terms of structured stimulation (Gottfried, 1984) – but also is devoid of love and affection, if not frankly abusive. Yet I have presented evidence from our own research to show that it is not necessary to seek examples of deprivation so extreme as an upbringing in a cellar or an old-fashioned foundling home to find retardation in linear growth in association with impaired cognitive development, including language. We have observed this association in a British inner-city preschool population, within the past decade.

A related issue, and one not explicitly addressed so far, is *by what mechanisms* are these features of children's development impaired in the first place? In other words, although it is easy to speak glibly of 'extreme deprivation' it is of both theoretical and practical interest to enquire – deprivation of what? These are complex issues and the answers are by no means clear cut. However, some pointers do seem indisputable .

First, it is most unlikely that either growth or language development is impaired primarily because of a lack of love, in the sense of an attachment relationship. The early views of Goldfarb (1944; 1945) and Bowlby (1951) have subsequently been disconfirmed, as lowered IQ and delayed language development do not result simply from the absence of a single stable adult attachment figure during early childhood (Tizard and Rees, 1975). Also, our own work on children's recovery from psychosocially induced short stature has indicated that, with respect to linear growth impairment, it is probably the *presence* of overt hostility and abuse that is largely responsible for the diminution in growth hormone secretion, rather than the *absence* of a strong attachment relationship. Children can show what appears to be reactive hypersecretion of growth hormone in hospital *despite* the absence of any special nursing arrangements (Stanhope et al., 1988). Just how the change in environment mediates this dramatic hormonal restitution is unknown, although clinical observations and some interesting recent work with rat pups (Schanberg and Field, 1987) and preterm neonates (Field et al., 1986; Scafidi et al, 1990) suggests physical contact may be a crucial element. The mechanisms inducing short stature in children who are *not* subject to abuse and neglect remain unclear: nutritional factors may have a role to play but this is not usually a straightforward example of chronic malnutrition (Skuse, 1989a).

What, then, are the minimum requirements for the normal acquisition of language? Language development is not retarded among children living in conditions of deprivation simply by a *lack* of stimulation; the quality as well as the quantity of input is of crucial importance. This matter can be demonstrated quite clearly by studying, for example, the development of language among the hearing children of deaf parents (see Schiff-Meyers, 1988) who can develop speech and language normally if exposed to minimal speech that is ordered into subject–verb–object relations, and also have exposure to television. A recent review of the subject concluded (Mogford and Bishop, 1988) that, for children living in conditions of relative socioeconomic adversity, *clinically* significant language impairment, as opposed to *statistically* significant impairment, is unlikely to be attributable to environmental impoverishment alone.

However, where there is associated abuse and neglect the following mechanism may be relevant: first, environmental stressors acting upon the abused and neglected children can limit lexical learning; secondly, the children may not be exposed to the variety of experiences and interaction necessary for the learning of new words; thirdly, the quality of parent–child interaction necessary for syntactic and morphological learning may be impaired (Blager and Martin, 1976; Allen and Oliver, 1982). It has even been proposed that a child's lack of language skills could exacerbate neglect by causing a failure of positive reinforcement of maternal approaches (Fox, Long and Langlois, 1988).

Recovery of language after it has been impaired because of an *extraordinary* degree of deprivation seems to be achieved, in most cases, by nothing more sophisticated than the opportunity for living in a normally stimulating home and forming emotional bonds to a caring adult. A caretaker's qualities of emotional availability, sensitive responsivity, encouragement and provision of perceptual stimulation known to be important for normal children's development (Dowdney, 1988, unpublished PhD thesis) are also the salient influences bearing on later learning and maturation in those unfortunate children. Interventions necessary to bring about improvement in the skills of relatively less deprived, but abused and neglected children, or those living in conditions of severe social disadvantage, probably need to be more structured; however, their trajectories of recovery are far less well documented.

The long-term outcome for the growth of abused and neglected children who remain with their families of origin, and for excessively short children living in our inner cities, is also an inadequately researched subject. What evidence we have suggests that without a radical change of environment there is unlikely to be any significant alteration in the trajectories of linear growth, which will continue to lie in the lower reaches of the normal range (Skuse, 1989c; Oates, Peacock and Forrest, 1985).

Finally, we are left with one last question. What is the evidence for 'sensitive periods' for physical growth and language skills, deprivation during which can lead to long-standing and possibly permanent detrimental consequences? This issue with respect to physical growth is easily answered; growth virtually ceases when a child enters puberty and the epiphyses of the long bones fuse (Tanner, 1989). The degree to which a successful 'catch-up' occurs depends on what duration of time the child's bones have available in which to grow before puberty supervenes, and how rapidly linear growth increases relative to this 'aging' of the bones. So long as maturation of the bones remains delayed, growth continues – it may go on for considerably longer than is usual in normal children.

The answer with respect to language is far less clear cut, and may differ according to how the question is phrased. In theory, there might be periods in early life during which *some* exposure to language (which may not necessarily be verbal) is essential or else no language facility can subsequently develop. Not surprisingly, we have very little data on which to test this hypothesis. Lenneberg (1967) may have been correct when he suggested that language acquisition must occur during the first 12 years if it is to proceed normally, but notwithstanding the evidence on the development of Genie (Curtiss, 1977) – another child brought up in conditions of extreme isolation – we just do not know. Given some degree of prior exposure before puberty, it seems likely that otherwise normal children can and do learn language very rapidly when their perceptual environment improves and they can engage in contingent interactions with a caretaker. Long-lasting detriment to cognitive development, including language skills, is unlikely to result directly from a lack of early perceptual experience. Yet there is some evidence suggestive of a 'sensitive period' from the work of Money and colleagues (1983) discussed earlier.

There are also meticulous studies by Tizard and her colleagues over the past 20 years and more of children who were raised in residential nurseries and then adopted, or who were restored to their families of origin. The essential finding relevant to this issue, which is rather similar to that reached by Money, is as follows. Studied up to the age of 16 years (Hodges and Tizard, 1989a), children who had been adopted before the age of 4 years had a far better chance of showing major IQ gains than those were were adopted later. There are a number of possible explanations: the first possibility is that the children were subject to selective placement (Tizard and Hodges, 1978); that is, the brighter children were perhaps more appealing to prospective adopters and so were adopted earlier. The evidence on that subject is equivocal. Secondly, children who were older when placed in their adoptive family may have spent less time than the relatively younger preschool children in interaction with their parents. Thirdly, such late-adopted children had spent a greater period of their early lives in institutions, which lacked the depth and range of everyday experience that would be associated with a family upbringing. Accordingly, it is possible that the later adopted children may have lacked the firm basis on which to build social relationships and profit from them to the same extent as those adopted earlier in life (Hodges and Tizard, 1989b). They may subsequently have failed to learn to the same extent from their environment; certainly there was evidence that many of those formerly institutionalised children were likely to have difficulties in social relationships which persisted right up until 16 years of age, not only within their families but also affecting relationships outside those families, with peers and adults. Those difficulties were more marked among the late-adopted than the early-adopted sample (Figures 3.6 and 3.7).

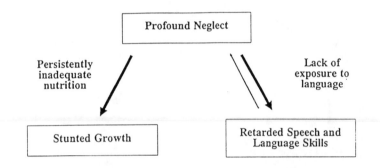

**Figure 3.6** Causal hypothesis on the relationship between impaired speech and language skills and retarded growth. Emphasis on environmental influences: neglect.

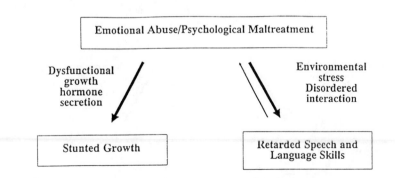

**Figure 3.7** Causal hypothesis on the relationship between impaired speech and language skills and retarded growth. Emphasis on environmental influences: abuse.

## Conclusions

I have presented a range of data showing that there does seem to be a link between impaired language development and impaired growth, in children growing up in conditions of relative deprivation, that is rather closer than one might expect by chance. Could they by any chance be related? There are four plausible possibilities for a causal relationship. The first and simplest is that, in a seriously neglectful environment their caretaking is relatively devoid of both adequate nutritional provision and an appropriate quality of linguistic stimulation. The association between the outcomes is due to their shared dependency on a common cause.

The second possibility is that a severely abusive environment

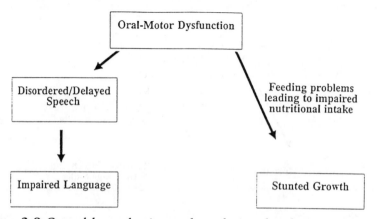

**Figure 3.8** Causal hypothesis on the relationship between impaired speech and language skills and retarded growth. Emphasis on intra-individual characteristics: dysfunctional oral–motor skills.

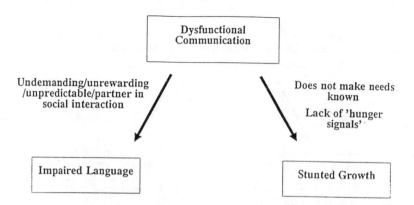

**Figure 3.9** Causal hypothesis on the relationship between impaired speech and language skills and retarded growth. Emphasis on intra-individual characteristics: dysfunctional communication skills.

interferes with the child's ability to learn, from whatever stimulation is available, and also – by some process we do not fully understand – cause retarded growth by interfering with growth hormone secretion. Again, the two outcomes are associated, due to a common cause.

Thirdly, the child may have some disorder of oral-motor functioning that interferes with the ability to feed adequately, and leads on to a speech problem which in turn impairs the acquisition of normal language skills (Figures 3.8 and 3.9). We have some evidence on this matter from our own research on oral-motor dysfunction in infants who fail to thrive (Mathisen, Skuse and Wolke, 1989).

Fourthly, the child may not possess a normal repertoire of communication skills, possibly because of brain damage, often because of what appears to be a normal variation in that repertoire of abilities that are necessary for adequate self-regulation. Such children may appear to be ideal babies; they are undemanding and easily soothed. They may be 'good sleepers' – indeed, one of their chief characteristics is that they sleep during, or even through, feeds (Reilly and Skuse, 1991). Because of their poor communication to the caregiver – either through unclear signals, or a lack of any signals at all, they may not be fed adequately – leading eventually to retarded growth, and they may also not elicit the quality in interaction in terms of dialogue that is essential for normal language acquisition (Stern et al., 1975). This group of children have been little studied so far, yet their condition may be the commonest of all. It is important to bear in mind that the degree to which their handicap affects developmental abilities depends crucially upon the sensitivity and responsivity of their caregiver.

In conclusion, the acquisition of language and the regulation of somatic growth seem to be linked in interesting and unexpected ways. We still have much to learn about the causal mechanisms that are responsible for this serendipitous observation. A greater understanding of these issues would be of considerable theoretical interest and practical significance, but might also illuminate developmental pathways that have hitherto barely been recognised.

## Acknowledgements

I am grateful to Jill Hodges for her advice and help in the planning of this paper, and to my assistant Jennifer Smith for her extraordinary skills in mastering arcane software during preparation of the manuscript.

## References

ALLEN, R.E. and OLIVER, J.M. (1982). The effects of child maltreatment on language development. *Child Abuse and Neglect*, 6, 299–305.

BLAGER, F.B. and MARTIN, H.P.. (1976). Speech and language of abused children. In: H.P. Martin (Ed.) *The Abused Child: A multidisciplinary approach to developmental issues and treatment,* pp. 83–92. Cambridge: Ballinger Publishing.

BOWLBY, J. (1951). *Maternal Care and Mental Health.* Geneva: World Health Organization.

CHERNOVA, T.V. (1990). Morbidity and physical development of children's homes residents. *Soviet Zdravookbr,* 7, 34–36.

CICCIETTI, D. and CARLSON, V. (1989). *Child Maltreatment.* Cambridge: Cambridge University Press.

CLAUSSEN, A.H. and CRITTENDEN, P.M. (1991). Physical and psychological maltreatment: relations among types of maltreatment. *Child Abuse and Neglect,* 15, 5–18.

CURTISS, S. (1977). *Genie: A psycholinguistic study of a modern-day 'wild child'.* London: Academic Press.

DOWDNEY, L. (1988). The parenting behaviour of women raised in institutions. University of London: PhD Thesis.

DOWDNEY, L., SKUSE, D., HEPTINSTALL, E., PUCKERING, C. and ZUR-SZPIRO, S. (1987). Growth retardation and developmental delay amongst inner-city infants. *Journal of Child Psychology and Psychiatry,* 28, 529–541.

FIELD, T.M., SCHANBERG, S.M., SCAFIDI, F., BAUER, C.R., VEGA-LARH, N., GARCIA, R., NYSTROM, J. and KUHN, C. (1986). Tactile/kinesthetic stimulation effects on preterm neonates. *Pediatrics,* 77, 654–658.

FOX, L., LONG, S.H. and LANGLOIS, A. (1988). Patterns of language comprehension deficit in abused and neglected children. *Journal of Speech and Hearing Disorders,* 53, 239–244.

GOLDFARB, W. (1944). Infant rearing as a factor in foster home replacement. *American Journal of Orthopsychiatry,* 14, 162–166.

GOLDFARB, W. (1945). Effects of psychological deprivation in infancy and subsequent stimulation. *American Journal of Orthopsychiatry,* 102, 18–33.

GOTTFRIED, A. (1984). *Home environment and early cognitive development.* New York: Academic Press.

HEPTINSTALL, E., PUCKERING, C., SKUSE, D., DOWDNEY, L. and ZUR-SZPIRO, S. (1987). Nutrition and mealtime behaviour in families of growth retarded children. *Human Nutrition: Applied Nutrition,* 41a, 390–402.

HODGES, J. and TIZARD, B. (1989a). IQ and behavioural adjustment of ex-institutional adolescents. *Journal of Child Psychology and Psychiatry,* 30, 53-76.

HODGES, J. and TIZARD, B. (1989b). Social and family relationships of ex-institutional adolescents. *Journal of Child Psychology and Psychiatry,* 30, 77–98.

KING, J.M. and TAITZ, L.S. (1985). Catch up growth following abuse. *Archives of Disease in Childhood,* 60, 1152–1154.

KOLUCHOVA, J. (1972). Severe deprivation in twins: a case study. *Journal of Child Psychology and Psychiatry,* 13, 107–114.

KOLUCHOVA, J. (1976). The further development of twins after severe and prolonged deprivation: a second report. *Journal of Child Psychology and Psychiatry,* 17, 181–188.

KOLUCHOVA, J. (1979). Lo sviluppo psichico di due gemmeli monozigotici a seguito di una grave e prolungata deprivazione. In: Cesa-Bianchi, M. and Poli, M. (Eds.), *Aspetti biosociali dello sviluppo. Vol 1: Aspetti medico-biologici.* Proceedings of the IVth ISSBD conference, Milan.

KOLVIN, I., MILLER, F.J.W., SCOTT, D., GATZANIS, S.R.M. and FLEETING, M. (1990). *Continuities of Deprivation?* Aldershot: Avebury.

LENNEBERG, E. (1967). *Biological Foundations of Language.* New York: John Wiley and Sons.

LYNCH, A., MITCHELL, L.B., VINCENT, E.M., TRUEMAN, M. and MACDONALD, L. (1982). The McCarthy Scales of Children's Abilities: a normative study on English 4 year olds. *British Journal of Educational Psychology*, **52**, 133–143.

MCCARTHY, D. (1972). *The McCarthy Scales of Children's Abilities*. New York: Psychological corporation.

MATHISEN, B., SKUSE, D. and WOLKE, D. (1989). Oral-motor dysfunction and failure to thrive amongst inner-city children. *Developmental Medicine and Child Neurology*, **31**, 293–302.

MOGFORD, K. and BISHOP, D. (1988). *Language Development in Exceptional Circumstances*. London: Churchill-Livingstone.

MONEY, J., ANNECILLO, C. and KELLEY, J.F. (1983). Growth of intelligence: failure and catchup associated respectively with abuse and rescue in the syndrome of abuse dwarfism. *Psychoneuroendocrinology*, **8**, 309–319.

OATES, R.K., PEACOCK, A. and FORREST, D. (1985). Long term effects of non-organic failure to thrive. *Pediatrics*, **75**, 36–40.

PREECE, M. and BAINES, J. (1978). A new family of mathematical models describing the human growth curve. *Annals of Human Biology*, **5**, 1–24.

REILLY, S. and SKUSE, D. (1991). Feeding practices and the growth of 'sleepy infants'. (in preparation).

ROSS, J.B. and MCLAUGHLIN, M.M. (Eds)(1949). Salimbene de Adam, Cronica, edited by F. Bernini (2 vols. Bari, 1942). I. 507. (translated) *The Portable Medieval Reader*, pp. 366–367, New York.

SCAFIDI, F.A., FIELD, T.M., SCHANBERG, S.M., BAUR, C.R., TUCCI, K., ROBERTS, J., MORROW, C. and KUHN, C.M. (1990). Massage stimulates growth in preterm infants: a replication. *Infant Behavior and Development*, **13**, 167–188.

SCHANBERG, S.M. and FIELD, T.M. (1987). Sensory deprivation stress and supplemental stimulation in the rat pup and preterm human neonate. *Child Development*, **58**, 1431–1447.

SCHIFF-MEYERS, N. (1988). Hearing children of deaf parents. In: Mogford, K. and Bishop, D. (Eds), *Language Development in Exceptional Circumstances*, pp. 47–61. London: Churchill-Livingstone.

SKUSE, D. (1985). Non-organic failure to thrive: a reappraisal. *Archives of Disease in Childhood*, **60**, 173–178.

SKUSE, D. (1989a). Emotional abuse and delay in growth. *British Medical Journal*, **299**, 113–115.

SKUSE, D. (1989b). Emotional abuse and neglect. *British Medical Journal*, **298**, 1692–1694.

SKUSE, D. (1989c). Psychosocial adversity and impaired growth: in search of causal mechanisms. In: Williams, P., Wilkinson, G. and Rawnsley, K. (Eds.), *The Scope of Epidemiological Psychiatry. Essays in honour of Michael Shepherd*, pp. 240–263. London: Routledge.

SKUSE, D., WOLKE, D. and REILLY, S. (1990). How often are failing to thrive infants abused or neglected? Presentation at the 62nd Annual Meeting of the British Paediatric Association, Warwick.

SPITZ, R.A. (1945a). Hospitalism: an inquiry into the genesis of psychiatric conditions in early childhood. *Psychoanalytic Study of the Child*, **1**, 55–74.

SPITZ, R.A. (1945b). Hospitalism: a follow-up report. *Psychoanalytic Study of the Child*, **1**, 113–117.

STANHOPE, R., ADLARD, P., HAMILL, G., AMOS, J., JONES, J., SKUSE, D. and PREECE, M. (1987). Physiological growth hormone (GH) secretion during recovery from psychosocial dwarfism. *Journal of Endocrinology*, **115**, Suppl 21.

STANHOPE, R., ADLARD, P., HAMILL, G., AMOS, J., JONES, J., SKUSE, D. and PREECE, M. (1988). Physiological growth hormone (GH) secretion during recovery from psychosocial dwarfism. *Journal of Endocrinology*, **28**, 335–339.

STERN, D., JAFFE, J., BEEBE, B. and BENNETT, S. (1975). Vocalizing in unison and in alternation: Two modes of communication within the mother–infant dyad. In: D. Aarsonson and R.W. Rieber (Eds), *Developmental Psycholinguistics and Communication Disorders*. New York: New York Academy of Sciences.

TAITZ, L.S. and KING, J.M. (1988a). A profile of abuse. *Archives of Disease in Childhood*, **63**, 1026–1031.

TAITZ, L.S. and KING, J.M. (1988b) Growth patterns in child abuse. *Acta Paediatrica Scandinavica* Supplement, **343**, 62–72.

TANNER, J.M., WHITEHOUSE, R.H. and TAKAISHI, M. (1966). Standards from birth to maturity for height, weight, height velocity, weight velocity: British children 1965. *Archives of Disease in Childhood*, **41**, 454–471.

TANNER, J. (1986). Growth as a target-seeking function. Catch-up and Catch-down growth in man. In: Falkner, F. and Tanner, J. (Eds), *Human Growth: A comprehensive treatise*, pp. 167–179. Plenum: New York.

TANNER, J.M. (1989). *Foetus into Man: Physical growth from conception to maturity*, 2nd edn. Ware: Castlemead Publications.

TERMAN, L.M. and MERRILL, M.A. (1960). *Stanford–Binet Intelligence Scale: Manual for the 3rd revision, form L-M*. Boston: Houghton Mifflin.

TIZARD, B. and REES, J. (1975). The effect of early institutional rearing on the behaviour problems and affectional relationships of four-year-old children. *Journal of Child Psychology and Psychiatry*, **16**, 61–74.

TIZARD, B. and HODGES, J. (1978). The effect of early institutional rearing on the development of eight-year-old children. *Journal of Child Psychology and Psychiatry*, **19**, 99–118.

WECHSLER, D. (1976). *Wechsler Intelligence Scale for Children – Revised* (manual). London: The Psychological Corporation.

ZDANSKA-BRINCKEN, M., GRODZKA, K., KURNIEWICZ-WITCZAKOWA, R., SZILAGYI-PAGOWSKA, I., ANTOSZEWSKA, A. and KOPCZYNSKA-SIKORSKA, J. (1983). Level and characteristics of the psychosomatic development of children from nurseries. *Probl-Med-Wieku-Rozwoj*, **12**, 7–26.

# Chapter 4
# Genetics and language disorder

MARCUS PEMBREY

## Introduction

The emergence of linguistic competence in a child is a wonderful thing to witness and, to elucidate the developmental brain processes that underlie this, must be one of the greatest challenges of human biology. From what we already know of mammalian developmental genetics, the sequential, coordinated action of a network of genes can be expected to play a central role in that element of brain development on which language acquisition will depend. Currently we have no idea which genes are involved or, equally important, how many alternative developmental routes will allow 'good enough' language and speech to emerge, albeit at a slower rate in some instances.

Given the evolutionary importance of speech for human survival and successful mating and parenting, it would be surprising indeed if compensatory mechanisms did not exist that would tend to mask genetic or acquired defects that interrupt just one of the regular developmental pathways. It follows that even complete loss of a gene function, such as would occur with deletion of much of its DNA sequence, could result in only a fairly subtle language deficit that would need detailed and expert testing to reveal. Appreciation of the consequences of these expected compensatory mechanisms is important for research planning. It is salutary to note that two years ago the 'received wisdom' was that the key mammalian genes concerned with the body plan (the so-called *Hox* genes) were so important that a deletion of any one of them would cause the early embryo to die. It was, therefore, considered futile and naive in the extreme to propose searching for deletions in the equivalent human *Hox* genes in infants with inherited multiple malformation syndromes. However, the new ability to actually 'knock out' a selected *Hox* gene in mouse embryos has revealed an example where knocking out one copy produces no discernable effect and knocking out both copies of the *Hox* 1.5 gene produces viable offspring with multiple malformations (Chisaka and Capecchi, 1991). Clearly, considerable compensatory mechanisms can exist. A developmental function may be so important that effective backup systems have evolved and, as a consequence, quite subtle neurological dysfunction may be due to substantial genetic defects. Some language and speech disorders could well fall into this category.

What with this buffering effect of the developmental network and the complex and confounding interactions between genetic and environmental influences, it is not surprising that it can be difficult to determine to what extent differences between children with and without a particular language disorder are due to differences in their genes – their DNA sequence.

The accumulating indirect evidence for genetic influences in speech and language disorders has been discussed in several reviews (Ludlow and Cooper, 1983; Bishop, 1987). Baraitser (1987) covers the topics he discussed at the first AFASIC conference in Reading, which include the empirical sibling recurrence risks for dyslexia and stuttering, as well as a discussion of selected genetic syndromes that feature speech and language problems. Radcliffe (1982) has reviewed speech and learning disorders in children with sex chromosome abnormalities. In this chapter I will explore a much more direct approach to genetic influences that has been made possible by the revolutionary developments in gene mapping and molecular genetics. The encouragement to do this comes from two sources; a remarkable family (G6393) that appears to have a dominantly inherited speech disorder (Hurst et al., 1990) and the recent advances in our understanding of the genetics of Angelman syndrome (Angelman, 1965), a mental retardation disorder in which speech is disproportionately affected (Robb et al., 1989).

## A Mutation that Specifically Affects Speech and Language Development?

In experimental animal work one would start to piece together the interacting components of a complex system by altering one component at a time and seeing what happens. Obviously in human biology the opportunities to use this approach are severely limited and, certainly where genetic factors are concerned, one has to rely on the discovery of a natural experiment where a mutation has produced a discrete and reproducible change in the function of the system as a whole. Given the complexity of language development and the expectation that compensatory systems would have evolved that could rescue development if one element failed, it was all the more surprising and exciting to discover family G6393. The substantial research programme that has begun on this family at the Institute of Child Health, London was a direct result of the AFASIC conference in Reading in 1987.

My colleague, Dr Baraitser, was approached after the conference by Elizabeth Auger of the Speech and Language Unit, Lionel Primary School in Middlesex, where several family members attended. The pedigree in Figure 4.1 comes from the paper Dr Hurst and Dr Baraitser wrote with Ms Auger, Ms Graham and Ms Norell of the Speech and Language Unit. It is because the family is so large that it raises the possibility of mapping and eventually defining this remarkable mutation. What must be remembered, if this were to be successful, is that it would define a monogenic language disorder, not 'a gene for speech' and certainly not '*the* gene for speech'. Just because the cause of a watch stopping can be simple, does not mean that the cause of it working is simple. However, characterising

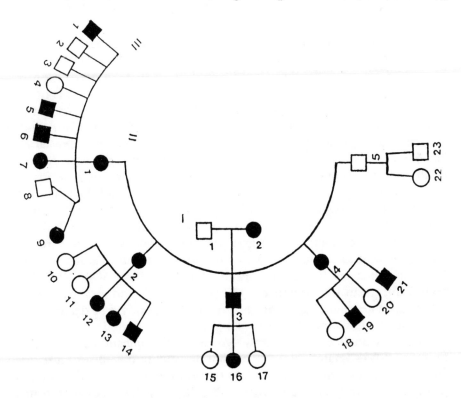

**Figure 4.1** Pedigree of family G6393 with filled symbols indicating affected individuals. □, ■, males; ○, ● females. Reproduced with permission from Hurst et al., 1990.

the G6393 family mutation would define a gene that is critically involved in language development. If the appropriate functioning of this gene did not represent a critical, almost pivotal, element in speech development, then its malfunction would not produce such a devastating effect so regularly. An understanding of when this gene is expressed during fetal and infant brain development, and in what cells, will open up a direct study of brain function in relation to speech and language. How good is the evidence that a dominantly inherited mutation is the cause of the language disorder in family G6393 and how discrete, characteristic and unusual is the language disorder? The answer to the first question depends on the answer to the second.

## The Language Disorder in Family G6393 and its Inheritance

At the time of referral to the Hospitals for Sick Children, Great Ormond Street/Institute of Child Health (HSC/ICH), seven members of the family were pupils at Lionel Primary School and other members of the family had been pupils in the past. Both sexes exhibited severe speech impairment with mispronunciation and agrammatism that rendered the children's utterances largely unintelligible. The designation of 16 of the family members as affected in the report of Hurst et al. (1990) – Figure 4.1 – was based on examination of six affected individuals in generation III and family reports of similar problems, supported by assessments of the staff of the speech and language unit in the other 10. Those designated unaffected attended normal schools and were reported to have normal speech and language development. Since that initial report, the family has been cooperating with an extensive series of psycholinguistic and neurological tests at the Institute of Child Health by a group comprising Dr Faraneh Vargha-Khadem, Dr Dick Passingham, Dr Paul Fletcher and Professor Brian Neville. To date, nine childen and four adults in three generations have been studied and the main features are as follows. They have an articulatory dyspraxia with relative preservation of receptive language and preserved input phonology in the absence of dysarthria, hearing loss or low intelligence. Using the WAIS-R/WISC-R scales, the mean performance IQ of these 13 affected members is 95 (80–112). With reference to the Hurst et al. (1990) pedigree designation, 15 of the 29 family members have been confirmed as definitely affected, 12 definitely unaffected, with only two children of questionable status at present. It is estimated by the ICH team that children with such a severe and unusual speech disorder would be very uncommon in the general population. In the face of this, the relatively clear-cut difference between affected and unaffected members and the occurrence of 15 definitely affected members out of 29 over three generations affecting both sexes equally, is highly indicative of autosomal dominant inheritance. In support of this, the unaffected male, II-5, has unaffected children. X-linked inheritance is not formally excluded because there has been no opportunity, so far, for male-to-male transmission.

Such a concentration of a rare distinct disorder in 15 members of one family makes polygenic and multifactorial inheritance very unlikely.

### The Strategy to Map the G6393 Mutation

The strategy for mapping the G6393 mutation is summarised in Table 4.1. The family is, *in theory*, large enough to allow mapping of the mutant gene to within a chromosomal region of about 5–10 centimorgans, assuming all the 26 relevant meioses are informative and no recombination is observed with a particular polymorphic marker. The prospects for such a mapping study are improving all the time with the development of new, simplified polymerase chain reaction-based techniques using sets of highly informative polymorphisms which arise in stretches of DNA containing variable numbers of tandem repeats of simple sequences, e.g. $(CA)_n$ (Weber and May, 1989).

It is essential to assign the phenotype *before* doing the linkage analysis, so there can be no possibility of being tempted to re-evaluate the phenotypic assignment of an individual who happens to be the only recombinant with the marker under study. If, after detailed evaluation of

**Table 4.1**

| The general gene mapping approach | Finding the mutant gene in family G6393 |
| --- | --- |
| 1. A clear-cut disorder (phenotype) | a. Characterise the speech/language disorder in family G6393 |
| 2. One or more large families where the disorder (or susceptibility to it) is inherited in a simple mendelian fashion | |
| 3. Test for co-inheritance with DNA sequences of known chromosomal location | b. Assign phenotypes and *then* map the mutation |
| 4. Map disorder to a chromosomal region | |
| 5. Build up a local physical map of overlapping fragments of DNA | |
| 6. Search for DNA sequences characteristic of genes coding for proteins | c. Select 'neurogenes' mapping to the region as candidate genes |
| 7. Test each candidate gene for appropriate expression | d. Test genes in the region for appropriate expression in fetal brain |
| 8. Compare the DNA sequence of normal controls and subjects | e. When the mutant gene is characterised, look for minor variations in language-delayed children |

the whole family, any individual remains unclassifiable, then that person would have to be left out of the analysis. If it were possible to map the G6393 mutation, the next problem is to discover the relevant gene in a DNA sequence of many megabases in length. The Human Genome Project and related research aimed at cloning genes expressed in fetal and adult brain will generate many 'long shot' candidates. However, those genes mapping to the same chromosomal region as the G6393 mutation will become serious candidates justifying extensive study. It should be emphasised that mapping and eventually defining the mutant gene is likely to take a very long time, although I believe it is achievable. At present we are at the stage of defining the phenotype and assigning family members as affected or not affected.

The whole mapping process would be enhanced if other families with *exactly* the same disorder were discovered. This in turn means the delineation of language disorders in detail becomes very important.

### The Problem of Genetic Heterogeneity

There are two broad types of genetic heterogeneity; so-called *allelic* heterogeneity, where different mutations can occur in the same gene (locus), and *locus* heterogeneity, where very similar disorders are due to mutations at entirely different gene loci, mapping to different chromosomal regions. In linkage studies, pooling pedigrees in which different gene loci are involved usually confounds the study, unless all the families are large. There is no way of knowing whether two mutations at different loci could produce exactly the same language disorder, although one can hope that differences would emerge if the disorder were dissected in enough detail. The dependence of gene mapping on such careful phenotypic analysis cannot be emphasised too strongly. It would be surprising if further families with a mutation at the same gene as in family G6393 did not exist. It may be that one or more of the four pedigrees described by Lewis (1990) will prove to be the same on detailed analysis. Mapping the G6393 mutation will immediately enable smaller families in which a language disorder is segregating to be classified into those that map to a different gene locus and those that are compatible with involvment of the G6393 gene locus. Once classified this way, useful discriminating features in phenotype between the two classes can be sought.

The problems posed by possible locus heterogeneity have been reviewed recently in connection with mapping apparently inherited forms of dyslexia (Smith et al., 1990). An earlier study had indicated that a mutation causing specific reading disability was located on chromosome 15 (Smith et al., 1983). However, an independent group was unable to confirm this linkage in Danish families with dyslexia (Bisgaard et al., 1987), although this does not necessarily mean that the earlier work was wrong. Locus genetic heterogeneity may exist and the matter needs to be resolved with further linkage studies on large families.

In summary, there seems little doubt that characterising the G6393 mutation would be of great interest from the standpoint of understanding the genetic influences on language and speech development. There are many different directions in which further research could go, including a search for DNA sequence variations in the gene in children with the commoner forms of specific developmental language disorder.

However, this gene hunt could take a long time. An alternative strategy is to assess whether any of the 'neurogenes' that have been cloned, or are likely to be discovered in the near future, can throw some light on the genetics of speech development. One such candidate is the gene involved in Angelman syndrome (AS). It is recognised, of course, that with the absent or near-absent speech set against a background of severe learning difficulties and other neurological deficits, interpretation of the developmental molecular genetics with respect to speech and language may be problematic. However, children with AS probably have sufficient preservation of general comprehension to allow some useful psycholinguistic analysis. Certainly these children present clinically with a very distinctive and unusual behavioural phenotype in which their speech problem appears disproportionately severe. Another reason for interest in the normal function of the gene that is mutant in AS children is that we now know it is subject to genomic imprinting, a recently recognised phenomenon of parental origin effect on gene expression. Genomic imprinting could be – and this is pure speculation – implicated in the genetics of social behaviour including language and speech development.

## Angelman Syndrome

Angelman syndrome was first described in 1965 by Harry Angelman (Angelman, 1965) who reported three children with severe mental retardation, no speech, jerky voluntary movements, ataxic gait, a seizure disorder and characteristic facial features. Children with AS also have a particularly happy disposition. In most cases the occurrence is sporadic, but several familial cases of AS have been documented and the recurrence risk, although low, is not negligible. High-resolution chromosome studies have revealed a de novo deletion of 15q11–13 in about half the sporadic cases (Kaplan et al., 1987; Magenis et al., 1987; Pembrey et al., 1989) whilst other patients, including all the familial cases to date, have normally appearing chromosomes (Knoll et al., 1990; Imaizumi et al., 1990).

There has been a long-standing interest in AS patients at the Institute of Child Health/Hospitals for Sick Children (ICH/HSC). Boyd, Harden and Patton (1988) described the characteristic EEG changes that are so helpful in confirming the diagnosis. Robb et al. (1989) described the clinical features of the first 36 AS patients in our series and noted that speech is absent or extremely limited. Scoring all the sounds that parents indicate are meaningful words, the maximum number observed in any child was six. This near absence of speech, even in teenage years after intensive training, has been confirmed by Dr Jill Clayton-Smith, who has now studied the clinical features of 84 individuals as part of the ICH/HSC ongoing research. To date there have been no detailed psycholinguistic data reported on children with AS. In an ICH/HSC pilot study (M. Ryan and N. Jolleff, personal communication) using the Bzoch–League Receptive Expressive Emergent Language Scales and a Modified Pre-verbal Communication Schedule of Kiernan and Reid, on 11 children ranging in age from 2;6 years to 15;3 years it was concluded that despite achieving a basic level of verbal comprehension the AS children rarely develop recognisable speech. Those that had learned Makaton signs largely used them for labelling or after a direct request to use them, but not for spontaneous communication. Ryan and Jolleff suggest that 'these children either have a motor planning problem which affects the development of speech and use of gesture and signing, or alternatively they have a fundamental problem of using communication for social interaction', but they recognise that a proper in-depth study is required to start to define the psycholinguistic and behavioural phenotype in this disorder.

## The Genetics of Angelman Syndrome

The genetics of AS is so remarkable that the neurodevelopment of this disorder is likely to be characterised in detail as part of the elucidation of how the normal gene at 15q11–13 functions. This gene is yet to be discovered, but it almost certainly will be in the next year or so.

The first hint of the unusual inheritance of the gene that is deleted or mutant in AS came from the observation that all the de novo 15q11–13 microdeletions were on the *maternally* derived chromosome 15 (Donlon, 1988; Knoll et al., 1989). In the ICH/HSC series, in collaboration with the cytogeneticist, Tessa Webb in Birmingham, we have shown to date that 29 out of 29 microdeletions are maternally derived. These data suggest that the normal gene is 'silenced' in some way when transmitted by the father, so a paternally derived mutation or de novo deletion confined just to the AS locus would have no effect on the child who inherited it.

(It happens that the gene locus for an entirely different mild/moderate mental retardation disorder, the Prader–Willi syndrome (PWS), is located very close to the AS locus and *paternally* derived microdeletions, including both the AS and PWS loci, will cause PWS without features of AS).

Final proof of this normal 'silencing' of the paternal gene at the AS locus comes from two sources. First, we observed (Malcolm et al., 1991) that two patients with AS and normal-looking karyotypes had inherited two intact chromosome 15s from father and none from mother, a phenomenon called uniparental disomy. Clearly, normal brain development cannot be rescued by the inheritance of two normal 15s from father. (A similar phenomenon, but the converse; namely, uniparental maternal disomy, has been observed in the non-deletion cases of PWS (Nicholls et al., 1989)). Secondly, Hamabe et al. (1991) have just reported a family where three affected AS siblings with normal-looking chromosomes do in fact have a tiny deletion at the DNA level within the 15q11–13 region of their maternally derived 15. Their mother, who is phenotypically normal, also has the DNA deletion and she herself inherited it from her own phenotypically normal father. Because she inherited it from her father, the gene would be normally silenced anyway, so the DNA deletion was inconsequential.

It is not known yet how many human genes show this parental origin effect on gene expression, but it is a phenomenon that can no longer be ignored when considering the interaction between genetic and environmental influences, particularly on an evolutionary timescale.

## Genomic Imprinting in Normal Development

There is currently great interest in the normal non-mutational modification of certain genes during egg and sperm formation, such that the gene from only one parent (and not both as is usually the case) is operational in the offspring. Of course, the 'imprint' to silence the gene from the other parent will need to be erased between generations if the gene is not to be eventually silenced completely, regardless of which parent transmits it.

Studies of genomic imprinting in the human are, as yet, very limited, but there is increasing information on imprinted loci in mice. Perhaps the most intriguing observation to date is that the *paternal* gene for the insulin growth factor II receptor (mouse chromosome 17) is the one that is silenced (Barlow et al., 1991) whereas for the insulin growth factor II itself (mouse chromosome 7) it is the *maternal* gene that is silenced (DeChiara, Robertson and Efstratiadis, 1991). Although IGFII is not the major ligand of the IGFII receptor, this observation still suggests that genomic imprinting is not just an incidental by-product of local chromatin structure but has some functional and therefore evolutionary significance in terms of development and metabolism.

It is perhaps worth adding, as an aside, for those who regard DNA sequencing as the worst form of reductionism, that human molecular genetics has been greatly illuminated by taking an evolutionary perspective. Molecular genetics regularly reveals links between humans and the other animals. As a short cut to knowing whether or not the DNA sequence in the test tube is an expressed gene of importance, the molecular geneticist will usually run a 'zoo blot'. This is an array of DNA fragments from different animals from fruit fly to human. If the particular DNA sequence has been conserved throughout a substantial period of evolution, it can be concluded that it 'does something important'. It will be worth remembering that any gene concerned rather specifically with language development might not be revealed by the 'zoo blot' screen although, knowing the propensity for evolutionary mechanisms to adapt what already exists for new purposes, it would be surprising if such genes did not have a counterpart in some other animals.

Returning to the phenomenon of genomic imprinting, I wish to conclude with some speculation on its possible evolutionary significance. The only reason that the silencing effect of some imprinting factor (presumably a DNA binding molecule) is known to operate at the Angelman syndrome gene locus during spermatogenesis, is because this does *not* happen during oogenesis. We can only observe the phenomenon because there is a *difference* in expression depending on the parental origin. It is possible that what we are seeing with genes showing a parental origin effect on their expression is not the whole story, but a 'window' on a general drift of some genes into inactivity regardless of which parent transmits them. Such genes would constitute a form of 'comatosed' genome – silent for a few or many generations before either accumulating disabling DNA mutations to be lost forever, or being recruited back into the active genome by a lifting of the imprint that had silenced them. Given that a molecular mechanism does exist for both selectively imprinting some genes and for erasure of this imprint between generations, there exists also the potential for a physiological adaptive process mediated through metabolic events that influences imprinting during gametogenesis. It has the potential to allow fine tuning of the organism's *active* genetic make up in response to environmental (and social) changes over several generations.

This system of silencing and recruiting, or perhaps some less extreme modulation of gene expression, could provide the basis for a relatively rapid evolutionary response; just what one might expect to be important for the emergence of social humans and, of course, language and speech development.

The above is just wild speculation. We know the AS locus is subject to imprinting, and mutations there have a marked effect on language and speech development amongst other things. However, the gene locus at which the G6393 mutation occurs does not appear to be imprinted, because transmission of the mutation from either parent results in an affected child. The genetic influences on language development can be expected to be complex and we know so little at present, but the application of the new techniques for mapping and defining mutations to the sort of families I have described is likely to be a fruitful way forward.

## References

ANGELMAN, H. (1965). Puppet children. *Developmental Medicine and Child Neurology*, 7, 681–688.

BARAITSER, M. (1987). Genetic aspects of speech disorders. *Journal of Tropical Pediatrics*, 33, 162–165.

BARLOW, D.P., STOGER, R., HERMAN, B.G., SAITO, K. and SCHWEIFER, N. (1991). The mouse insulin-like growth factor type 2 receptor is imprinted and closely linked to the Tme locus. *Nature*, 349, 84–87.

BISGAAD, M. L., EIBERG, H., MOLLER, N., NIEBUHR, E. and MOHR, J. (1987). Dyslexia and chromosome 15 heteromorphisms: negative lod score in Danish material. *Clinical Genetics*, 32, 118–119.

BISHOP, D.V.M. (1987). The causes of specific developmental language disorder ('Developmental Dysphasia'). *Journal of Child Psychology and Psychiatry*, 28, 1–8.

BOYD, S.G., HARDEN, A. and PATTON, M.A. (1988). The EEG in early diagnosis of Angelman's (happy puppet) syndrome. *European Journal of Pediatrics*, 147, 503–513.

CHISAKA, O. and CAPACCHI, M. R. (1991). Regionally restricted developmental defects resulting from targeted disruption of the mouse homoebox gene *hox*-1.5. *Nature*, 350, 473–479.

DECHIARA, T.M., ROBERTSON, E.J. and EFSTRATIADIS, A. (1991). Parental imprinting of the mouse insulin-like growth Factor II gene. *Cell*, 64, 849–859.

DONLON, T.A. (1988). Similar molecular deletions on chromosome 15q11.2 are encountered in both the Prader–Willi and Angelman syndromes. *Human Genetics*, 80, 322–328.

HAMABE, J., KUROKI, Y., IMAIZUMI, K., SUGIMOTO, T., FUKUSHIMA, Y., YAMAGUCHI, A., IZUMIKAWA, Y. and NIIKAWA, N. (1991). DNA deletion and its parental origin in Angelman syndrome patients, *American Journal of Medical Genetics*, 41, 64–68

HURST, J.A., BARAITSER, M., AUGER, E., GRAHAM, F. and NORELL, S. (1990). An extended family with a dominantly inherited speech disorder. *Developmental Medicine and Child Neurology*, 32, 352–355.

IMAIZUMI, K., TAKADA, F., KUROKI, Y., NARITOME, K., HAMABE, J. and NIIKAWA, N. (1990). Cytogenetic and molecular study of Angelman syndrome. *American Journal of Medical Genetics*, 35, 314–318.

KAPLAN, L.C., WHARTON, R., ELIAS, E., MANDELL, F., DONLON, T. and LATT, S.A. (1987). Clinical heterogeneity associated with deletions in the long arm of chromosome 15: report of 3 new cases and their possible genetic significance. *American Journal of Medical Genetics*, 28, 45–53.

KNOLL, J.H.M., NICHOLLS, R.D., MAGENIS, R.E., GRAHAM, J.M., LALANDE, M. and LATT, S.A. (1989). Angelman and Prader-Willi syndromes share a common chromosome deletion but differ in parental origin of the deletion. *American Journal of Medical Genetics*, 32, 285–290.

KNOLL, J.H.M., NICHOLLS, R.D., MAGENIS, R.E., GRAHAM, J.M., KAPLAN, L. and LALANDE, M.

(1990). Angelman syndrome: three molecular classes identified with chromosome 15q11–13 specific DNA markers. *American Journal of Human Genetics*, 47, 149–155.

LEWIS, B.A. (1990). Familial phonological disorders: four pedigrees. *Journal of Speech and Hearing Disorders*, 55, 160–170.

LUDLOW, C. L. and COOPER, J. A. (Eds.) (1983). *Genetic Aspects of Speech and Language Disorders*. New York: Academic Press.

MAGENIS, R.E., BROWN, M.G., LACY, D.A., BUDDEN, S. and LA FRANCHI, S. (1987). Is Angelman syndrome an alternate result of del(15)(q11-q13)? *American Journal of Medical Genetics*, 28,829–838.

MALCOM, S., CLAYTON-SMITH, J., NICHOLS,.M., ROBB, S., WEBB, T., ARMOUR, J. A. L., JEFFREYS, A. J.and PEMBREY, M. E.(1991). Uniparental disomy in Angelman syndrome. *Lancet*, 337, 694–697.

NICHOLS, R.D., KNOLL, J.H.M., BUTLER, M.G., KARAN, S. and LALANDE, M. (1989). Genetic imprinting suggested by maternal heterodisomy in non-deletion Prader–Willi syndrome. *Nature*, 342, 281–282.

PEMBREY, M.E., FENNEL, S.J., VAN DEN BERGHE, J., FITCHETT, M., SUMMERS, D., BUTLER, L., CLARKE, C., GRIFFITHS, M., THOMPSON, E., SUPER, M. and BARAITSER, M. (1989). The association of Angelman's syndrome with deletions within 15q11–13. *Journal of Medical Genetics*, 26, 73–77.

RADCLIFFE, S.G. (1982). Speech and learning disorders in children with sex chromosome abnormalities. *Developmental Medicine and Child Neurology*, 24, 80–84.

ROBB, S.A., POHL, K., BARAITSER, M., WILSON, J. and BRETT, E.M. (1989). The 'happy puppet' syndrome of Angelman – review of the clinical features. *Archives of Disease in Childhood*, 64, 83–86.

SMITH, S.D., KIMBERLING, W.J., PENNINGTON, B.F. and LABS, H.A. (1983). Specific reading disability: identification of an inherited form through linkage analysis. *Science*, 219, 1345–1347.

SMITH, S.D., ENNINGTON, B.F., KIMBERLING, W.J. and ING, P.S. (1990). Familial dyslexia: use of genetic linkage data to define subtypes. *Journal of the American Academy of Childhood Psychology*, 29, 204–213.

WEBER, J.L. and MAY, P.E. (1989). Abundant class of human DNA polymorphisms which can be typed using the polymerase chain reaction. *American Journal of Human Genetics*, 44, 388–396.

# Chapter 5
# Language delay and social development

MICHAEL RUTTER, LYNN MAWHOOD AND PATRICIA HOWLIN

Over the years, specific developmental language disorders have been conceptualised in a variety of different ways. At one time, neurologists tended to extrapolate from acquired language disorders as seen in older children or adults, and terms such as developmental aphasia came to be in vogue (Benton, 1964). Then, those with a paediatric background pointed out various crucial differences and the concept of an isolated delay in a specific developmental function, namely language, came to the fore (Ingram, 1959). There was some dispute between those who viewed the delay as a manifestation of an impaired maturation of a specific brain system and those who conceptualised the delay as an extreme, but essentially non-pathological, end of a continuum of normal variation in the pace of language development (Bishop and Rosenbloom, 1987). A byproduct of that particular controversy was the parallel dispute over whether the language was deviant or just delayed (Menyuk, 1977). The matter cannot be said to be resolved but there has been a tendency to favour the delay concept (Bishop and Edmundson, 1987b). However, two trends have raised questions on the issue. First, numerous studies have shown the high frequency with which language delay is associated with later socioemotional, behavioural and educational problems (Rutter and Mawhood, 1991). Why does this happen? It has been argued that the problems are merely a reflection of neurodevelopmental immaturity, and not psychopathology as it is ordinarily conceptualised (Tallal, Dukette and Curtiss, 1989), but are they?

Second, the notion that the delay solely and specifically involves language has been called into question by the evidence that there are associated cognitive problems of various sorts (Tallal, 1985). Thus, Tallal and colleagues have shown that the language problems tend to be associated with perceptuomotor impairments and especially with difficulties in temporal sequencing (see Tallal, 1985). Similarly, Bishop and Edmundson (1987b) noted close links between motor and language development, and Stark, Mellits and Tallal (1983) found that the degree of perceptuomotor impairment predicted language outcome. Children with developmental language disorders have also been shown to have deficits in representational or symbolic thinking (Morehead and Ingram, 1973, Kahmi et al, 1984), associative imagery and short-term memory (Eisenson, 1968; Masland and Case, 1968; Menyuk, 1969, Graham, 1974), auditory processing (Tallal and Piercy, 1975, Tallal, 1976) and sequencing (Efron, 1963; Poppen et al, 1969). It is striking that these findings on the broader cognitive deficits often associated with specific developmental language disorders (at least of the more severe types) have become established at a time when researchers in the field of normal language development have shown the considerable extent to which language develops *independently* from general intelligence (Bates, Bretherton and Snyder, 1988). Does this mean that specific developmental language disorders (SDLD) represent a *dis*continuity with normality? Probably it does in some instances. Certainly, it is known that a few cases are due to chromosomal anomalies (Walzer, 1985) and other clear-cut medical abnormalities. But known causes account for a very small proportion of cases of SDLD; what about the remainder? It is clear that some examples of delay in acquiring spoken language represent no more than extreme normal variations. Just as normal children vary greatly in the age when teeth erupt or puberty is reached, so children are likely to vary in the age when they first begin to speak. At the other extreme, it is evident from the associated neurodevelopmental and cognitive problems that some cases of marked language delay represent pathology. Few would doubt that there are these two broad classes of language delay, but their differentiation at an individual level has proved somewhat difficult (Stark, Mellits and Tallal, 1983, Bishop and Rosenbloom, 1987).

One way of tackling this issue is to examine the long-term course of development with reference, not just to the progression in language, but more especially to associated problems in socioemotional and behavioural development and to their predictors. That is the purpose of this chapter. In planning better services for young people with specific developmental language disorders, we need to know the range of psychological problems that they face as they grow up. However, if we are to devise effective preventive and therapeutic interventions, we must also determine the mechanisms involved. As we shall see, that is a more difficult challenge but, nevertheless, it is one that cannot be shirked.

## Follow-up into Middle Childhood

Let us begin with the findings on studies that have followed groups with SDLD into middle childhood (Rutter and Mawhood, 1991). The best data are provided by Bishop and her colleagues (Bishop and Edmundson, 1987a, b; Bishop and Adams, 1989), who undertook a prospective longitudinal study of 87 4-year-old children with a marked language impairment, together with a cross-sectional control group. All but two of the 87 children had a score on at least one language measure below the 3rd percentile, with no more than one score (out of 9) above the 10th percentile.

Thus, they comprised a group with a clinically significant severe delay; 68 of the 87 children had a non-verbal IQ in the normal range on the Leiter scale. The first striking finding is that, at follow-up at 5½ years, nearly half (44%) no longer met the criteria for severe language impairment. This 'good outcome' group continued to progress, and at a further follow-up at 8 years of age their language skills were only very slightly below those of controls.

We may infer that many of these children had experienced a delay in language development that was essential normal – an extreme, it is true, but one with virtually full catch-up in language functions. The next question is what features served to characterise this 'good outcome' group. The findings showed that many of these children had a pure phonological impairment and the remainder had a mild impairment of a narrow range of language functions.

If we turn now to the characteristics of those with a persistent language deficit, it is evident that they showed a severe and broad language impairment, involving receptive language and also associated perceptuomotor abnormalities. Other studies have also shown that a poor prognosis is associated with qualitatively abnormal features of language, with associated neurodevelopmental abnormalities and with an impairment of general intelligence.

The next issue concerns the general finding that children with developmental language disorders have a substantially increased risk for later reading difficulties (Rutter and Mawhood, 1991). Six main queries arise from this finding: (a) whether the scholastic risk is mainly a function of general intellectual impairment or a specific language deficit; (b) whether the risk is specifically for reading difficulties or more generally for a broad range of scholastic problems; (c) which types of speech/language deficit lead to the greatest scholastic risk; (d) whether the scholastic risk associated with a specific language disorder differs in degree or pattern from that associated with developmental disorders of non-language functions (such as motor or perceptual skills); (e) following the last point, whether the risk stems from the fact that language as such is impaired or from neurodevelopmental or cognitive deficits that may underlie the language disorder; and (f) whether the risk applies only when there is persistent language impairment or whether it applies also to transient language difficulties.

The Bishop follow-up findings (Bishop and Adams, 1990) are important in showing that the increased rate of scholastic difficulties did not apply to the 'good outcome' SDLD group whose language had reached normal levels by age 8 years; that the main association was between language impairment and reading comprehension; but that there were non-verbal as well as verbal deficits at age 8; and that there was little, if any, scholastic deficit associated with pure phonological difficulties. In short, these findings, as well as those from other studies, indicate that the factors associated with a less good language outcome also predict scholastic difficulties.

Both epidemiological and clinical studies are agreed that children with SDLD also show a raised frequency of socioemotional and behavioural problems (Rutter and Mawhood, 1991). There does not appear to be anything diagnostically specific about the associated psychiatric problems but the main increase seems to be in the domains of anxiety, social relationships and attention-deficit problems rather that in conduct disturbance or antisocial behaviour. One might expect these difficulties to be maximal in early childhood when the language impairment is at its worst, but that does not seem to be the case. The few follow-up data suggest that the psychopathological problems tend to increase rather than diminish as the young people grow older (Baker and Cantwell, 1987a; Cantwell et al., 1989).

The psychopathological risk is greater if language delay is accompanied by lower than average intelligence, but it is still substantial even when the IQ is normal. The findings from studies indicate that, for SDLD children of normal IQ, the risk is greatest when there is a deficit in spoken language and not just an articulation or phonological problem; when language comprehension is affected and when there is some impairment in cognitive functioning (Baker and Cantwell, 1987b; Beitchman et al., 1989a, b). The implication, once more, is that the psychological sequelae are greatest in the case of language disorders that seem more than just extremes of the normal range and hence that the risk may not stem directly from the language delay as such. That inference clearly raises the need to compare the sequelae of developmental disorders of language with other types of developmental disorder – such as the 'clumsy child' syndrome. Curiously, there is a lack of any direct comparisons of this kind.

There has been scarcely any research into the mechanisms involving these psychopathological associations (Howlin and Rutter, 1987). However, several possibilities may be suggested. Thus, it could be that in some cases common antecedents might explain both the language delay and the associated socioemotional and behavioural problems. These could include temperamental difficulties, neurodevelopmental impairment and psychosocial disadvantage, for example. Alternatively, it could be that difficulties in communication or language oddities increase the risk of social rejection. Or, again, the scholastic problems that often follow language delay could constitute the mediating variable through the stresses accompanying educational failure. With the most severe language disorders, there is also the possibility that both the language delay and the psychological difficulties stem from a broader cognitive deficit, albeit one that has not substantially depressed overall intellectual functioning as reflected in the IQ.

## Follow-up into Adult Life

Before discussing these alternatives further, let me turn to what is known on adult outcome for the group most at risk; namely children with severe developmental disorders of receptive language. In that connection, it is necessary to rely on our own findings.

Our strategy involved a focus on outcome in early adult life (at a mean age of 24 years) of matched groups of SDLD and autistic boys of normal non-verbal intelligence, first studied in the early school years (at the mean age of 7½ years) (Bartak, Rutter and Cox, 1975; Cox et al., 1975). There was an intermediate assessment in middle childhood (at a mean age of 9½ years) (Cantwell et al., 1989). We built in the comparison with autism because this was a condition that involved a comparable degree of language impairment in early childhood but which stood out at that age as very different in terms of socioemotional and behavioural features. All children with a hearing loss of 40 decibels or more were excluded on the basis of testing in early childhood; however, at follow-up it was clear that three SDLD men had a major hearing loss and they have been excluded from the findings presented here. The comparison, then, is between 19 men with autism and 20 with SDLD. The follow-up assessment included standardised interviews with parents and the subjects themselves, together with standardised observations and systematic psychological testing.

In turning now to the follow-up findings, let us start with the outcome on language, as it was the delay in language acquisition that provided the starting point for the selection of the sample (Table 5.1). All of the SDLD men had gained conversational language but four autistic men remained without any useful language. Moreover, as was the case when they were young, abnormal language features in terms of echoing and stereotyped qualities were characteristic of autism but not at all of

**Table 5.1** Abnormal language features in autistic and SDLD men

|                                        | Autism | SDLD  |
|----------------------------------------|--------|-------|
| Negligible speech                      | 4      | 0     |
| Echolalia                              | 7      | 0     |
| Stereotyped phrases                    | 8      | 0     |
| Prosodic oddities (marked)             | 12 (7) | 9 (1) |
| Lack of vocal expressiveness (marked)  | 9 (5)  | 6 (0) |
| Total                                  | 19     | 20    |

SDLD. On the other hand, although marked prosodic oddities and marked lack of vocal expressiveness were largely confined to the autistic sample, mild abnormalities in these features were quite common in the SDLD group.

Overall, the SDLD group had made more progress in language than the autistic group (Figure 5.1). The autistic group had a more severe initial deficit in receptive language but this did not account for the outcome difference between the groups. As observed, 13 of the 19 autistic men showed markedly poor conversational skills at follow-up, whereas that was so for only one of the 20 SDLD men. Nevertheless, half the SDLD group has some difficulties in conversation. Only about a third of both groups had fully adequate expressive language functioning. The differences between the groups on receptive and written language were, however, striking. Of the SDLD group 80% were thought to have normal receptive language skills; nearly twice the rate in the autistic group. Psychometric testing showed the same difference. On the picture vocabulary test the autistic group had a mean standard score of 44 compared with 67 in the SDLD group. However, as with most measures, it was striking that the standard deviation was greater in the autism group. As a reflection of that fact, the autistic group included many more with very low scores; thus there were 69% of the autistic group with age equivalents below 10 years compared with 21% in the SDLD group. The autistic group was similarly much more impaired on the Oral Comprehension test. Note, however, that the SDLD group were particularly poor in their written communication, actually worse than the autistic group. It is of interest that, although the SDLD group were originally identified in early childhood in terms of their particularly poor receptive language skills, this was their most satisfactory language function in early adult life.

At the time the groups were selected (when the subjects were fairly young), it was a requirement that they all have a non-verbal IQ of 70 or greater. Over the course of the follow-up, both groups showed a mean

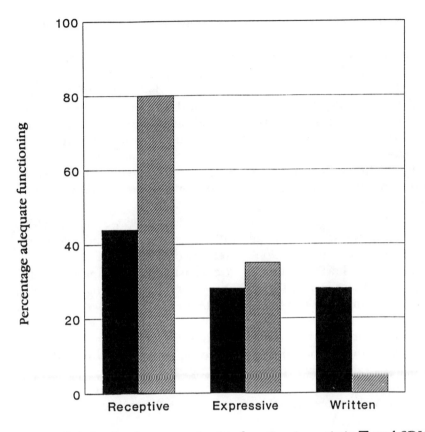

**Figure 5.1** Vineland communicative function in autistic ■ and SDLD ▨ men.

drop of 10–11 points. In most cases the first test was the WISC and the last the WAIS-R, so that the drop was not explicable in terms of a major change in test content.

Although both groups showed a mean drop in Wechsler performance IQ, their cognitive pattern at follow-up was not the same (Table 5.2). To some extent, this was evident in the overall scores on different tests. In the autistic group, there was a greater gap between the WAIS verbal IQ and the Ravens IQ; 21 points as against 11. At all time points, the Ravens Matrices provided the highest IQ score in the autistic group. Note, too, that again the spread of scores in the autistic group tended to be greater, although only markedly so for verbal IQ.

The pattern of performance subtests on the WAIS-R at follow-up also differentiated the groups, (as it had done similarly when they were first assessed). In the SDLD group the means for all subtests were at much the same level whereas the autistic group showed greater scatter. As found in previous studies, scores were highest on block design and object assembly and lowest on picture arrangement and picture completion.

There was no difference between the groups in attainment in reading, spelling, and arithmetic. In both groups, there were some men who achieved scores at the ceiling of the tests (15–17 years) but about half scored at below the 10 year level. Also in both groups, there was no association between non-verbal tests and attainment, and there was a substantial association with WAIS verbal IQ at follow-up. The groups differed, however, with respect to picture vocabulary. In the autistic group, both in childhood and adult life, this showed a substantial association with the composite attainment level (split into 8 years or under, over 8 years up to 12 years, and over 12 years).

Although the two groups were comparable at follow-up in overall IQ level and in scholastic attainments (with the autistic group actually somewhat superior in final educational level – two having gone to university, against zero in the SDLD group), the autistic group showed a much worse employment history (Table 5.4). Fourteen of the 19 had never had a paid job, against only two of the 20 SDLD men. However, only just over a third of the SDLD group had experienced regular paid employment. The majority had been in and out of work, without anything regular.

The continuing handicaps of the autistic men were also evident in their living arrangements (Figure 5.3). Over half were in some form of residential care and only 16% were living independently. Only one SDLD man was in residential care but over half were still living with

**Table 5.2** WAIS-R and Ravens' IQ for autistic and SDLD men

|  | WAIS verbal Mean (s.d.) | WAIS performance Mean (s.d.) | Ravens' Mean (s.d.) |
|---|---|---|---|
| Autism (*n*=19) | 73.3 (21.7) | 82.8 (13.1) | 94.6 (16.8) |
| SDLD (*n*=19) | 75.3 (7.8) | 78.4 (10.4) | 86.1 (14.5) |

**Table 5.3** Cognitive measures and friendships in autistic and SDLD men (ANOVA)

|  | Autism F value (*P*) | SDLD F value (*P*) |
|---|---|---|
| WAIS verbal | 16.2 (0.0005) | 2.6 (ns) |
| Picture vocabulary | 22.1 (0.0001) | 1.4 (ns) |
| Composite scholastic attainment | 9.1 (0.005) | 3.5 (ns) |

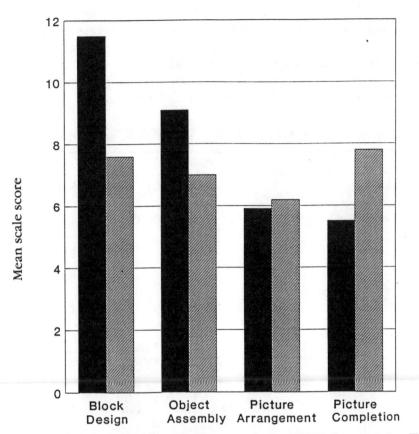

**Figure 5.2** Pattern of performance subtests WAIS for autistic ■ and SDLD ▨ men.

their parents – a surprisingly high proportion considering that they were in their mid 20s.

Table 5.5 shows the level of social competence at follow-up another way, in terms of the Vineland daily living skills scores. The SDLD men were average but the autistic men had a mean score of only 65 – over 30 points lower. Again there was a difference between the groups in the association with other variables. In the autistic group daily living skills

**Table 5.4** Employment history of autistic and SDLD men

|  | Autism (n=19) | SDLD (n=20) |
|---|---|---|
| Regular paid employment | 2 | 7 |
| In and out of work; not regular | 1 | 11 |
| No paid employment ever | 14 | 2 |
| Still in further education | 2 | – |

were strongly associated with language level, as assessed on the Vineland, whereas there was no such association in the SDLD group. However, in neither group did the language scores (on the Picture Vocabulary test) when the children were first assessed predict daily living skills at follow-up.

**Table 5.5** Vineland daily living skills scores for autistic and SDLD men

|  | Autism | SDLD |
| --- | --- | --- |
| Mean (s.d.) | 65.1 (35.0) | 99.2 (15.0) |
| Association composite language level F value (P) | 19.23 (0.0005) | 0.83 (ns) |

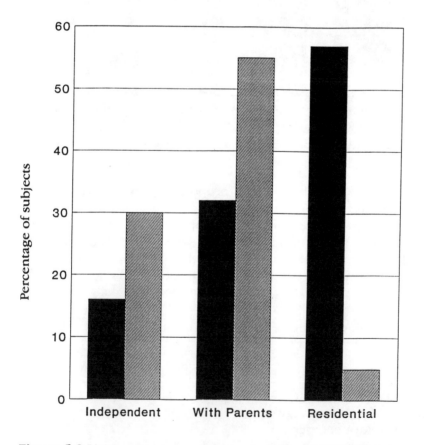

**Figure 5.3** Living arrangements for autistic ■ and SDLD ▨ men.

Finally, let us turn to the socioemotional functioning of the groups in early adult life. Various aspects of non-verbal communication were assessed as part of systematic observations using the Autism Diagnostic Observation Schedule (Lord et al., 1989) (Table 5.6). The autistic men stood out as obviously odd in terms of their lack of effective well integrated use of smiling and facial expression; three quarters showed deviance on these features and half markedly so. Marked abnormalities in these domains did not occur in the SDLD men but some oddities were noted in an appreciable minority.

Using a standardised interview with subjects and parents, the subjects' social relationships were assessed in some detail. The main findings are briefly summarised in Table 5.7. The great majority (15/19) of the autistic men continued to show major problems in this domain, having had neither a close friendship nor a love relationship. The SDLD men were functioning rather better so that, for example, four were married and two others had had a close heterosexual relationship. Nevertheless, it was striking that one-third had never had either a close friendship or a love relationship, and a further third had had only a close friendship but no love relationship.

**Table 5.6** Non-verbal communication in autistic and SDLD men

|  | Autism (n=18) | | SDLD (n=18) | |
| --- | --- | --- | --- | --- |
|  | Odd | Markedly deviant | Odd | Markedly deviant |
| Smiling | 13 | 9 | 3 | 0 |
| Facial expression | 14 | 8 | 7 | 0 |
| Non-verbal-language linkage | 14 | 9 | 3 | 0 |

**Table 5.7** Friendships and love relationships in autistic and SDLD men

|  | Autism (n=19) | SDLD (n=17) |
| --- | --- | --- |
| Close friendships and love relationships | 1 | 5 |
| Close friendships only | 3 | 6 |
| Neither | 15 | 6 |

**Table 5.8** Leisure activities outside the home environment in autistic and SDLD men

|  | Autism (*n*=18) % | SDLD(*n*=20) % |
|---|---|---|
| Engages regularly in range of leisure activities on own initiative | 28 | 30 |
| Some spontaneous leisure activities | 11 | 40 |
| Few spontaneous adult-type interests | 6 | 25 |
| Leisure activities arranged by others | 56 | 5 |

Much the same pattern of differences was seen with respect to leisure activities (Table 5.8). Over half of the autistic men seemed unable to organise their own leisure and had this organised for them by other people; this applied to only one SDLD man. At the other extreme, just over a quarter of both groups regularly engaged in a range of appropriate leisure activities that they organised for themselves. However, the SDLD group showed substantial limitations in their leisure life, two-fifths had rather limited activities and a quarter showed few spontaneous adult-type interests. For example, three spent hours watching the traffic, another went to bus stations to collect bus numbers and another with a special interest in buses frequently went off on bus journeys on his own.

Table 5.9 shows the association between cognitive measures and social functioning as indexed by close friendships at follow-up. In the autistic group, the WAIS verbal IQ, Picture Vocabulary score, and scholastic attainment were all strongly associated with social functioning, whereas there was a zero relationship in the SDLD group.

In conclusion, let us bring the findings together in relation to the questions raised earlier on the nature of specific developmental language disorders and on the mechanisms involved in the socioemotional sequelae. As we have seen, it is striking that these extended right into early adult life.

Before making any inferences on SDLD, the findings on autism may be summarised. In spite of the men's relatively normal level of non-verbal intellectual functioning, the follow-up showed extensive evidence of continuing handicaps in language, communication, daily living skills, scholastic attainment, socioemotional expressiveness and social relationship. Moreover, it was clear that there were quite strong interconnections between the autistic men's language and social functioning. It seems reasonable to suppose that cognitive deficits may well serve as a link between the two. Autism, therefore, constitutes a pervasive developmental disorder with problems in both the cognitive and social arenas that continue into adult life.

What about SDLD? The findings showed an interesting pattern of similarities and differences. The group was chosen to represent a severe, but supposedly specific developmental disorder of receptive and expressive language. All the SDLD men gained conversational language and a few showed fully normal language functioning in adult life; however, the group as a whole continued to show impairments in language, albeit not quite the same as those in autism. Stereotyped repetitive utterances and other gross abnormalities in the form of spoken language did not occur. On the other hand, prosodic oddities and a lack of vocal expressiveness were both evident in about half the group, although not so severe as in the autism group. Our analyses to date have not covered pragmatic aspects of language (Bishop and Adams, 1989) but it is clear that some of the SDLD men showed abnormalities in this domain. It remains to be determined whether or not these are associated with the social impairments.

The findings on cognitive performance provide both parallels and contrasts with autism. In both groups, there was a drop of 10–11 points in non-verbal IQ in spite of the marked improvements in language functioning. Together with the extensive evidence from other studies, this points to the presence of cognitive deficits that extend beyond language per se. Although the most obvious, and most severe, handicap in SDLD concerns language it cannot be regarded as a pure and simple language delay.

**Table 5.9** Cognitive measures and scholastic attainment in autistic and SDLD men (ANOVA)

|  | Autism F value ($P$) | | SDLD F value ($P$) | |
|---|---|---|---|---|
| **Childhood** | | | | |
| Picture vocabulary | 10.15 | (0.005) | 0.55 | (ns) |
| Ravens | 1.59 | (ns) | 0.11 | (ns) |
| **Adulthood** | | | | |
| Picture vocabulary | 21.68 | (0.0001) | 2.60 | (ns) |
| WAIS verbal | 13.68 | (0.0005) | 11.35 | (0.001) |
| WAIS performance | 2.52 | (ns) | 3.46 | (ns) |

While that seems clear, the mechanisms involved in the social impairments persisting into adult life remain uncertain. The finding that these have continued long after conversational language has been acquired suggests that it is implausible that the explanation lies mainly in terms of a psychological response to communication limitations as such. If that were the case, improvement with age should have occurred and greater accompanying emotional disturbance might have been expected. Neither was found. Nevertheless, it is also evident that, although all the SDLD men had acquired conversational language, in most cases their language functioning was not normal. Their mean standard score on the picture vocabulary test was only 67; they were particularly poor in written communication and their scholastic attainments were low. It would seem reasonable to suppose that these continuing cognitive and language limitations might have played a role in the men's impaired social relationships. However, in striking contrast to the findings in the autistic group, no association was found between these cognitive and language measures and the quality of social relationships. Of course, so far, only a limited range of cognitive and language functions have been examined. The social risks might stem from pragmatic aspects of language rather than comprehension; or from metacognitive rather than cognitive deficits, that is from limitations in the ability to appreciate and anticipate what other people are likely to be thinking and feeling in social situations. Such abilities were examined in one study of language-impaired children (Leslie and Frith, 1988) and no deficit was found. However, the test employed had quite a low ceiling and it is too early to conclude that there are no limitations in this cognitive domain. It is obvious that we have a lot yet to learn about the basis of the social relationship difficulties experienced by many adults with a severe developmental disorder of receptive language and the topic should have a high priority for future research.

In the meanwhile, it is important in the planning of services that we recognise that the difficulties experienced by young people with serious SDLD extend well beyond language and often include substantial problems in social relationships. In seeking to provide effective interventions to foster better social functioning we need to evaluate what we do in order that we may learn, not only which interventions are beneficial, but why and how they bring about gains so that an increased understanding of the processes involved may enable us to develop more effective methods of helping in the future.

## Acknowledgements

The research reported in this chapter constitutes part of Lynn Mawhood's PhD project. Support was generously provided by the John D. and Catherine T. MacArthur Foundation.

# References

BAKER, L. and CANTWELL, D. (1987a). Comparison of well, emotionally disordered and behaviorally disordered children with linguistics problems. *Journal of the American Academy of Child and Adolescent Psychiatry*, **26**, 193–196.

BAKER, L. and CANTWELL, D. (1987b). A prospective psychiatric follow-up of children with speech/language disorders. *Journal of the American Academy of Child and Adolescent Psychiatry*, **26**, 546–553.

BARTAK, L., RUTTER, M. and COX, A. (1975). A comparative study of infantile autism and specific developmental receptive language disorder. I. The children. *British Journal of Psychiatry*, **126**, 127–145.

BATES, E., BRETHERTON, I. and SNYDER, L. (1988). *From First Words to Grammar: Individual Differences and Dissociable Mechanisms*. Cambridge: Cambridge University Press.

BEITCHMAN, J., HOOD, J., ROCHUN, J., PETERSON, M., MANTINI, T. and MAJUMDAR, S. (1989a). Empirical classification of speech/language impairment in children I. Identification of speech/language categories. *Journal of the American Academy of Child and Adolescent Psychiatry*, **28**, 112–117.

BEITCHMAN, J., HOOD, J., ROCHUN, J. and PETERSON, M. (1989b). Empirical classification of speech/language impairment in children II. Behavioral characteristics. *Journal of the American Academy of Child and Adolescent Psychiatry*, **28**, 118–123.

BENTON, A. (1964). Developmental aphasia and brain damage. *Cortex*, **1**, 40–52.

BISHOP, D. and ADAMS, C. (1989). Conversational characteristics of children with semantic–pragmatic disorder. II What features lead to a judgement of inappropriacy? *British Journal of Disorders of Communication*, **24**, 241–263.

BISHOP, D. and ADAMS, C. (1990). A prospective study of the relationship between specific language impairment, phonological disorders and reading retardation. *Journal of Child Psychology and Psychiatry*, **31**, 1027–1050.

BISHOP, D. and EDMUNDSON, A. (1987a). Language-impaired 4-year olds: distinguishing transient from persistent impairment. *Journal of Speech and Hearing Disorders*, **52**, 156–173.

BISHOP, D. and EDMUNDSON, A. (1987b). Specific language impairment as a maturational lag: evidence from longitudinal data on language and motor development. *Developmental Medicine and Child Neurology*, **29**, 442–459.

BISHOP, D. and ROSENBLOOM, L. (1987). Childhood language disorders: classification and overview. In: Yule, W. and Rutter, M. (Eds.), *Language Development and Disorders*, pp 16–41. London: MacKeith Press.

CANTWELL, D., BAKER, L., RUTTER, M. and MAWHOOD, L. (1989). Infantile autism and developmental receptive dysphasia: a comparative follow-up into middle childhood. *Journal of Autism and Developmental Disorders*, **19**, 19–32.

COX, A., RUTTER, M., NEWMAN, S. and BARTAK, L. (1975). A comparative study of infantile autism and specific developmental receptive language disorders. II. Parental characteristics. *British Journal of Psychiatry*, **126**, 146–159.

EFRON, R. (1963). Temporal perception, aphasia and deja vu. *Brain*, **86**, 403–424.

EISENSON, J. (1968). Developmental aphasia (dyslogia). A postulation of a unitary concept in the disorder. *Cortex*, **4**, 184–200.

GRAHAM, N. (1974). Response strategies in the partial comprehension of sentences. *Language and Speech*, **17**, 205–221.

HOWLIN, P. and RUTTER, M. (1987). The consequences of language delay for other aspects of development. In: Yule, W. and Rutter, M. (Eds.), *Language Develop-*

*ment and Disorders*, pp 271–294. Oxford: MacReith Press.

INGRAM, T. (1959). Specific developmental disorders of speech in childhood. *Brain*, 82, 450–467.

KAHMI, A., CATTS, H., ROENIG, L. and LEWIS, B. (1984). Hypothesis testing and non-linguistic symbolic abilities in language impaired children. *Journal of Speech and Hearing Disorders*, 49, 169–176.

LESLIE, A.M. and FRITH, U. (1988). Autistic children's understanding of seeing, knowing and believing. *British Journal of Developmental Psychology*, 6, 315–324.

LORD, C., RUTTER, M., GOODE, S., HEEMSBERGEN, J., JORDAN, H., MAWHOOD, L. and SCHOPLER, E. (1989). Autism diagnostic observation schedule: A standardized observation of communication and social behavior. *Journal of Autism and Developmental Disorders*, 19, 185–212.

MASLAND, M. and CASE, L. (1968). Limitations of auditory memory as a factor in delayed language development. *British Journal of Disorders of Communication*, 3, 139–142.

MENYUK, P. (1969). *Sentences Children Use. Research monograph no. 52*, Cambridge MA: MIT Press.

MENYUK, P. (1977). *Language and Maturation*. Cambridge, MA: MIT Press.

MOREHEAD, D. and INGRAM, D. (1973). The development of base syntax in normal and linguistically deviant children. *Journal of Speech and Hearing Research*, 16, 330–352.

POPPEN, L., STARK, J., EISENSON, J., FORREST, T. and WERTHEIM, G. (1969).Visual sequencing performance of aphasic children. *Journal of Speech and Hearing Research*, 12, 288–300.

RUTTER, M. and MAWHOOD, l. (1991). The long-term psychological sequelae of specific developmental disorders of speech and language. In: Rutter, M. and Casaer, P. (eds.), *Biological Risk Factors in Childhood Psychopathology*. Cambridge: Cambridge University Press.

STARK, R., MELLITS, E. and TALLAL, P. (1983). Behavioral attributes of speech and language disorders. In: Ludlow, C. and Cooper, J. (Eds), *Genetic Aspects of Speech and Language Disorders*, pp. 37–52. New York and London: Academic Press.

TALLAL, P. (1985). Neuropsychological foundations of specific developmental disorders of speech and language: implications for theories of hemispheric specialisation. In: Cavenar, J. Jr. (Ed.), *Psychiatry:* Volume 3, pp. 1-15. Philadelphia: Lippincott.

TALLAL, P. (1976). Rapid auditory processing in normal and disordered language development. *Journal of Speech and Hearing Research*, 19, 561–571

TALLAL, P. and PIERCY, M. (1975). Developmental aphasia: the perception of brief vowels and extended stop consonants. *Neuropsychologica*, 12, 83–93.

TALLAL, P., DUKETTE, D. and CURTISS, S. (1989). Behavioral/emotional profiles of preschool language-impaired children. *Development and Psychopathology*, 1, 51–67.

WALZER, S. (1985). X chromosome abnormalities and cognitive development: implications for understanding normal human development. *Journal of Child Psychology and Psychiatry*, 26, 177–184.

# Part II

# Brain, Cognition and Language Impairment

# Chapter 6
# Brain injury and language impairment in childhood

DOROTHY M. ARAM

## Introduction

Study of the language development of young, brain-lesioned children has afforded an opportunity to address two issues central to the understanding of normal and disordered child language. The first issue concerns the degree of brain specialisation for language present in very young children and the degree to which language functions may reorganise, or are said to be 'plastic' if damaged early in life. By studying the language abilities of children who have sustained focal brain injury early in development in comparison to peers who have not sustained brain lesions, much can be learned relative to the degree to which language can develop in brain-lesioned children, the degree to which lateralised brain lesions (i.e. left versus right hemisphere involvement) are differentially related to language abilities, and the importance of other variables on eventual language performance, such as actual sites of brain involvement or the age at which injury was sustained.

While these and other questions related to brain and language relationships early in development have prompted many of the neurolinguistically oriented studies of children with brain lesions, study of these children also provides an avenue for addressing the neurological basis of developmental language disorders. Indeed, it is this latter issue that initially prompted my work involving children with lateralised brain lesions. Having had a long-standing interest in the biological basis of developmental language disorders, study of children with focal brain lesions, particularly those with focal left hemisphere lesions, permitted an opportunity to test the assumption that at least some developmental language disorders were attributable to left hemisphere dysfunction. By analogy to acquired aphasia in adults, it has long been presumed that developmental aphasia also was attributable to left hemisphere abnormalities. Through comparing the language abilities of children with verified focal brain lesions to that of children with language disorders but no verified brain lesions, similarities and dissimilarities could be drawn between their language deficits and inferences regarding common causality could be made.

The data presented here, then, address both of these issues: the degree of early brain specialisation versus reorganisation possibly following early lateralised brain lesions; and the parallels and implications for children with developmental language disorders but no known brain lesions. At the onset I want to acknowledge that during the past 10 years, several groups of investigators have begun to study language among children with lateralised brain lesions, including the important early work of Brian Woods (Woods and Teuber, 1978; Woods and Carey, 1979), Maureen Dennis' pivotal work with hemispherectomied children (Dennis and Kohn, 1975, Dennis and Whitaker, 1976; Dennis, Lovett and Wiegel-Crump, 1981) and a now growing group of investigators who have concentrated on children with lateralised brain lesions, Faraneh Vargha-Khadem (Vargha-Khadem, O'Gorman and Watters, 1985), Daria Riva (Riva et al., 1986), Isabelle Martins and Jose Ferro (Ferro et al., 1982; Martins, Ferro and Trindade, 1987), and Elizabeth Bates and colleagues in San Diego (Marchman, Miller and Bates, 1991; Thal et al., 1992). In the discussion that follows, I make no attempt to summarise in a comprehensive manner the important contributions of these other investigators. Rather I will be drawing principally from the series of studies my colleagues and I in Cleveland have undertaken since 1981. Throughout these studies our primary aims have been to describe the aspect of language under examination in comparison to carefully matched control subjects, and to relate language performance among the lesioned subjects to the variables of lesion laterality, site of lesion within a hemisphere and age of lesion onset. To date we have explored a number of areas beyond oral language, including reading abilities, mathematical performance, verbal and non-verbal memory, intelligence, central auditory functions, and hand and foot growth. Here, the discussion will be limited to studies of oral language including syntax, the lexicon, and phonology. Data also will be presented relative to these children's ability to process rapidly changing auditory stimuli and to mechanisms of reorganisation of language functions following left lesions.

## Subjects

Given that the data presented will largely be based on the children studied at Rainbow, these subjects will first be described in some detail. Since 1981 we have been involved in an ongoing NIH-supported study of the language and learning sequelae of children with unilateral brain lesions. During that time we have continued to add children to our study and have lost a few due to death or, in several instances, to the development of a seizure disorder necessitating use of anticonvulsants, in which case the children continued to be followed, but were reclassified into a non-focal brain involvement group. All lesioned children admitted into our study have met strict inclusion criteria; in fact, many children seen initially have not been entered into the study because they have failed to meet inclusion requirements. Inclusion criteria included:

1. Presence of a static, unilateral left or right vascular lesion as evidenced by the clinical neurological examination and initially a computed tomography (CT) scan, followed by a magnetic resonance imaging (MRI) scan for all but a few patients who could not undergo MRI scans (due to pacemakers, surgical clips or other counter-indications). Therefore, children have been excluded if they presented:
   (a) identified or suspected non-focal involvement, including those in whom lesions were sustained secondary to trauma, tumor or systemic infections;
   (b) ongoing seizure disorders, requiring anticonvulsant therapy; and
   (c) lack of observable lesions on CT or MRI scans.

2. Evidence of normal neurological and behavioural development prior to lesion onset for all patients sustaining lesions after the perinatal period, and no evidence of genetic or other neurological problems. Thus children have been excluded with:
   (a) neonatal complications beyond congenital heart disorders, such as prematurity, respiratory distress syndrome, asphyxia;
   (b) identified or suspected genetic syndromes, such as trisomy 21; and
   (c) abnormal motor, mental, or social development prior to lesion onset per parent report or chart review.

At present we have 32 left-lesioned and 17 right-lesioned children enrolled in the study. In the studies reported here, having been undertaken over a 10-year period, not all children have participated in all studies due to the age requirements for administration of some of the measures and the number and ages of the children enrolled at the time in which the study was conducted. Of the left-lesioned children, current age range is 1;3 years to 22;8 years with a mean age of 11;6 years. Fourteen sustained pre- or perinatal lesions (usually porencephalic cysts), with the latest lesion onset occurring at 15;11 years of age with a mean age of lesion onset at 3;4 years. Among the right-lesioned children, the youngest is currently 2;6 years, the oldest is 23;5 years and the mean age is 9;6 years. Eight right-lesioned subjects sustained perinatal lesions, and the oldest sustained lesion onset at 9;8 years of age with a mean lesion onset of 1.76 years. The older mean age of onset for the left-lesioned children is predominantly the result of five left-lesioned children all sustaining lesions after 10 years of age. Among the left-lesioned subjects there is a higher proportion of boys than girls (20:12) and among the rights the gender distribution is closely comparable, with eight boys and nine girls. Social class status for the lefts is somewhat more advantaged (2.12) than for the rights (mean Hollingshead score of 2.53). The majority of children experienced cerebrovascular accidents (11 lefts, 8 rights) usually secondary to congenital heart disorders, with other aetiologies including pre- or perinatal insults (14 lefts; 8 rights); arteriovenous malformations (4 lefts; 0 rights); and other causes, e.g. complications of complex migraine (3 lefts, 1 right).

Given the fact that the left and right lesioned groups were not comparable in age, sex, and social class, we have not been able to compare left- and right-lesioned children directly. Rather, each child has been individually matched to a neurologically normal child selected from children seen at our hospital with congenital heart disorders, since the majority of lesioned children had underlying congenital heart disorders. Control subjects, therefore, were selected on the basis of age, gender, race; socio-economic status using the Hollingshead 4-factor index; and arterial blood oxygen saturation level, with lesioned children who do not have congenital heart disorders matched only to acyanotic control children, and lesioned children with congenital heart disorders matched as closely as possible by arterial oxygen saturation levels.

Although all lesioned children identified during the acute period following lesion onset were followed at regular intervals (typically 1 month, 6 months and 1 year post-lesion onset and thereafter seen twice a year for additional studies), and we have reported case studies of some of these children during the more acute recovery period (Aram et al., 1983; Meyers, Hall and Aram, 1990), children were not included in group studies until at least 1 year had elapsed. Thus, the findings reported below reflect these children's ability at long-term follow-up as opposed to acute symptomatology. These then were the children who have served as subjects in the series of language studies conducted at Rainbow which will now be summarised.

## Language Abilities Among Children with Left or Right Brain Lesions

*Syntax*

*Spoken Syntax.* Surprisingly few reports of the connected spoken language of children with lateralised brain lesions have appeared. Several studies of children with acquired left (De Renzi and Vignolo, 1962; Alajouanine and Lhermitte, 1965; Dennis, 1980; Cranberg et al.,1987; Fletcher and Levin, 1988) and occasionally right brain lesions (Guttmann, 1942; Carter, Hohenegger and Satz, 1982) report mutism acutely and telegraphic expressive language during early recovery. Although Woods and Carey (1979) administered a sentence completion task to their 27 left-lesioned subjects and Kiessling et al. (Kiessling, Denckla and Carlton, 1983) administered the Binet Sentences, other than an occasional case report (e.g. Dennis, 1980), there have been no studies of connected spoken language of children with lateralised brain lesions.

Therefore, one of the earliest studies we undertook, based on only eight left and eight right-lesioned children, analysed the syntax of these children's spontaneous language (Aram, Ekelman and Whitaker, 1986). At the time this study was undertaken the left-lesioned children were between 2 and 8 years of age and the right-lesioned children were between 1;6 and 6 years of age. Numerous analyses of the spontaneous language samples were undertaken including calculating the mean length of utterance, the percentage of simple and complex sentences (including embeddings and conjunctions) attempted and the percentage correct, the Developmental Sentence Complexity score and subscores for pronouns, main verbs, interrogative reversals, wh-question and negatives, and the mean grammatical number and error rate. Although none of the children would be considered to be clinically aphasic at the time of test, left-lesioned subjects were found to perform more poorly than controls on most measures of simple and complex sentence structures. In contrast, right-lesioned subjects performed similarly to controls on these measures except for a tendency to make more errors in simple sentence structures. Although the differences between lesioned and control subjects were small, they consistently favoured left controls as being superior to left-lesioned subjects. The fact that right-lesioned children, whose intelligence indices were within normal limits but significantly lower than right controls, rarely differed from right controls on these syntactic measures was also notable. The left-lesioned group's achievement in syntax evidences the marked development, recovery and presumed reorganisation possible following left lesions in young children; yet in comparison to left controls and the absence of difference between right lesioned and control subjects, these findings evidence a specialised role of the left hemisphere in the development of spoken syntax in young children.

*Syntactic Comprehension.* We have conducted two studies addressing syntactic comprehension with our lesioned groups. The first reported these groups' performance on the *Revised Token Test* (RTT: McNeil and Prescott, 1978), which was selected from the array of *Token Test* versions due to the number of exemplars for each syntactic form assessed, and the scoring format which permitted qualitative scoring of correct and incorrect responses. Although there had been several previous reports of Token Test performance by left brain-lesioned children (Woods and Carey, 1979; Rankin, Aram and Horwitz, 1981; Ferro et al., 1982; Vargha-Khadem et al., 1985), none had evaluated the relative contribution of memory load versus syntactic comprehension to the results obtained. Our study included 17 left-lesioned children and their controls and 11 right-lesioned children (Aram and Ekelman, 1987). Overall, left-lesioned children performed significantly less well than left controls with particularly notable deficits on subtests IV to VIII. These differences, however, appeared to be related to the memory demands of these subtests rather than the admittedly limited syntactic elements assessed by the RTT. Right-lesioned subjects tended to perform more poorly than right controls, although these differences were not significant nor readily related to either the memory or specific linguistic structures assessed. This study, then, suggested a differential effect of left lesions on RTT performance, yet memory rather than syntactic demands may have been primary in contributing to these differences.

A more recent study involving these same children was carried out by Julie Eisele (Eisele, 1991). Fourteen left and 10 right lesioned children were compared with control subjects on their ability to judge the truth of embedded complements in sentences like 'Max remembered that he locked the door' and 'Max remembered to lock the door?' Sentences varied according to the type of matrix verb (know, remember or forget), the presence or absence of syntactic and/or lexical negation, and the syntax of the embedded complement (tensed or untensed). The results revealed hemispherical differences in syntactic, semantic and pragmatic language competence. The left-lesioned subjects failed to make use of the syntactic contrasts to judge truth-values, while right-lesioned subjects demonstrated a deficit in making use of certain types of lexical–semantic and pragmatic information. Although the data continue to be limited, these two studies suggest that even early in life the left hemisphere appears to have a special role in the comprehension of connected language that appears to be dependent upon syntactic aspects. In addition, Eisele (1991) demonstrated for the first time that, similar to what has been reported for adults, children with right hemisphere lesions also have difficulty comprehending connected language, due, at least in part, to pragmatic and lexical–semantic deficits.

## Lexical Abilities

Several investigators have addressed naming abilities among left or right-lesioned children (Woods and Carey, 1979; Kiessling, Denckla and Carl-ton, 1983; Vargha-Khadem et al., 1985), suggesting that both left- and right- brain-lesioned children may have persistent, albeit subtle, deficits in naming. We have attempted to extend these findings in two studies. The first of these studies examined lexical retrieval in response to semantic, visual and phonemic (rhyming) cues, using the Word-Finding Test, developed by Wiegel-Crump and Dennis (1984), and the Rapid Automatized Naming Task developed by Denckla and Rudel (1976). Nineteen left-lesioned and 13 right-lesioned children were included in this study (Aram, Ekelman and Whitaker, 1987). On the Word-Finding Test, left-lesioned subjects were significantly slower in response time than left controls when given semantic and visual cues and made more errors when given rhyming cues. On the Rapid Automatized Naming Task, left-lesioned subjects were significantly slower than left controls in naming all semantic categories, including colours, numbers, objects and letters. In contrast, right-lesioned subjects responded as or more quickly than did right controls in all cued conditions and yet tended to produce more errors than their controls. Increased latency of naming response was not associated with any particular lesion site in the left hemisphere, nor were there differences in lexical retrieval for children sustaining left lesions before versus after one year of age.

In a second study just completed (Eisele and Aram, 1992), we examined the relationship between left- and right-lesioned children's ability to comprehend lexical items, as assessed by the *Peabody Picture Vocabulary Test – Revised* (PPVT-R), and their ability to name lexical items, as measured by the *Expressive One-Word Picture Vocabulary Test* (EOWPVT). Unlike the normal control subjects, both the left- and right-lesioned children performed less well on the PPVT-R than on the EOWPVT, and both lesioned groups performed significantly worse than controls on the PPVT-R, but not on the EOWPVT. Among left-lesioned children, the higher a child's performance on the PPVT-R the higher the performance on the EOWPVT, resulting in smaller differences between the two measures. Among right-lesioned children, the PPVT-R scores remained relatively constant, with no score above the 50th percentile; thus, increases in the EOWPVT correlated with larger differences between the receptive and expressive lexical measures. These findings provide evidence that both the left and the right hemisphere contribute critically to the development of lexical comprehension in young children.

*Phonology*

Quite surprisingly, beyond case studies describing phonemic paraphasia (Visch-Brink and Sandt-Koenderman, 1984; Van Hout, Evrard and Lyon, 1985), little comment has been directed to the phonological production or articulatory abilities of children with lateralised lesions. The reports available are contradictory. Alajouanine and Lhermitte (1965) reported that when lesions occurred before 10 years of age, disorders of articulation were always present. Hecaen (1976) also stated that articulatory disorders were common when lesions were sustained before 10 years of age, and were observed following either left or right hemisphere lesions. More recent reports, however suggest that articulatory disorders are not common following lateralised lesions in children. For example Cranberg et al. (1987) noted that only one of eight children with acquired aphasia presented dysarthria. Kershner and King (1974) likewise found articulation errors to be no more common among left or right hemiplegic children than among controls.

Recently, Shriberg and Aram (1992) completed an exhaustive study of the phonology of the children followed at Rainbow. Based on narrow transcriptions of connected speech samples adhering to transcription conventions developed by Shriberg (Shriberg and Kent, 1982; Shriberg, Kwiatkowski and Hoffmann, 1984) and utilising the computer based analyses provided by PEPPER (Shriberg, 1986), speech production profiles of left-lesioned, right-lesioned and non-focal-lesioned children were compared to control subjects. Lesioned subjects had significantly lower speech production scores than did controls. Of the lesioned subjects 17% met criteria for clinical involvement compared with 3% of the control subjects. Speech status, however, was not significantly related to lesion laterality, age of lesion onset, site of lesion or gender. Although the brain-lesioned children as a group did present greater speech involvement than did controls, differences were small, few presented clinically significant involvement, and error patterns were similar to those observed in children developing speech normally or with speech delays of unknown origin. Unlike the majority of studies involving other aspects of language reported above, differences also were not significantly associated with lesion laterality. Two additional studies, although not directly bearing on any single aspect of language, are relevant to further discussion of the parallels between acquired and developmental language disorders in children, and will be summarised below.

**Auditory Temporal Perception**

Tallal (Tallal and Piercy, 1973; Tallal, 1976; Tallal, et al., 1980; Tallal, Stark and Mellits, 1985a) has presented evidence suggesting that children with developmental language disorders are specifically impaired in their ability to discriminate and sequence rapidly presented verbal and non-verbal stimuli. Inferring from studies of adults with left hemisphere lesions who, likewise, are unable to discriminate and sequence rapidly presented verbal and non-verbal stimuli (Tallal and Newcombe, 1978) it has been suggested that children with developmental language disorders who fail these tasks, also must have damage to the dominant cerebral hemisphere (Tallal, Stark and Mellits, 1985a, b; Tallal, 1987).

To test this inference, Tallal's task, the Repetition Task (Tallal and Piercy, 1973; Tallal, 1976) was administered to 20 left- and 12 right-lesioned children and their controls (Aram and Ekelman, 1988). Unlike adults with left hemisphere injury or children with developmental language disorders, neither left- nor right brain-lesioned children differed significantly from the control subjects. Since these results contrast with previous reports of impaired spoken syntax and lexical retrieval among many of the same left-lesioned children, we suggested that the higher level language deficits observed in these left-lesioned children could not be attributed to difficulty in analyses of the acoustic stimuli. These data also suggested that difficulty performing the Repetition Task could not be assumed to be related to left hemisphere lesions in children.

**Hemispheric Reorganisation of Language Functions**

Finally, there has been considerable speculation, although little actual data, relative to how and why children recover language functions more rapidly and completely than do adults with similar lesions. Several mechanisms, largely based on animal studies, have been proposed as providing the neurological basis for recovery or reorganisation of functions, yet very limited study has involved young children with lateralised brain lesions (Aram and Eisele, 1991). Probably the mechanism most frequently credited with a role in recovery is 'functional substitution', where it is speculated that 'uncommitted' portions of the same or contralateral hemisphere assume the displaced function. Too often it is somewhat glibly stated that the contralateral hemisphere 'takes over' functions of the hemisphere dominant for that function if damaged early in life. Yet, it must be reiterated that there is very little evidence that this actually occurs for language functions when injury is sustained in childhood. This assumption has largely been based on results of intracarotid amobarbital testing (WADA) to determine hemispheric lateralisation of language and memory functions before surgical resection for uncontrolled seizure disorders (e.g. Rasmussen and Milner, 1977). Yet even these studies of individuals with long-standing diffuse brain involvement demonstrate that the majority of individuals with left hemisphere lesions retain left hemisphere dominance for language, with a small proportion having some degree of bilateral contribution. Language restricted to the right hemisphere, however, is rarely borne out by the data (Loring et al., 1990).

Using what would appear to be a powerful but yet largely unexplored tool for studying hemispheric organisation of language functions following lateralised brain lesions in children, we undertook a study using evoked potentials (Papanicolaou et al., 1990). The paradigm used involved use of a probe-evoked technique which consisted of recording evoked potentials to a repetitive probe stimulus (a 500 Hz tone burst or strobe flash) presented during a control condition, and then again when subjects were engaged in a language or visuo-spatial task. The dependent measure was the amplitude of the evoked potential to that probe stimulus recorded from surface electrodes over the left and right hemispheric sites. For the verbal experimental task, we used a phonemic identification task, asking our 14 left-lesioned children and their controls to indicate by lifting both index fingers when they heard /br/, /p/ or /m/ from a tape-recorded list of unrelated words. The visual task involved a mental rotation task in which the subjects were asked to indicate if pairs of block designs presented in different orientations were the same (indicated by lifting the right index finger) or different (indicated by lifting the left index finger). In contrast to adult recovered aphasics previously studied with the identical task, in our study the children with left-hemisphere lesions displayed the normally expected pattern of predominant left-hemisphere engagement in the language (phonemic identification) task and right-hemisphere engagement in the visuo-spatial task. These data therefore suggested that, at least for the aspects of language examined here, phonemic identification, language restitution and development involved intrahemispheric, rather than interhemispheric, functional reorganisation.

## Summary and Implications for Children with Developmantal Language Disorders

In summary, across a range of language tasks including spoken syntax, syntactic comprehension, and lexical naming and retrieval, left-lesioned children as a group have presented consistent yet very mild deficits in abilities in comparison with normally developing children. Similar differences were not observed between right-lesioned children and their controls on the majority of these tasks; however, among right-lesioned children, lexical deficits in comprehension of single words were found, in addition to some preliminary data suggesting lexical and pragmatic deficits in comprehension of connected sentences. These findings, while suggesting some degree of lateralisation of early brain specialisation for different aspects of language, also attest to the marked recovery and presumed reorganisation of language abilities in young children in comparison with adults with similar brain lesions. What implications, then, do these data have for children with developmental language disorders? Before suggesting some admittedly speculative implications, it may be well to keep in mind that the findings reported here are at long-term follow up, typically involve children well beyond the preschool years, and do not address acute symptomatology or the longitudinal course of development and recovery. In young lesioned children, we frequently observe delayed onset of language, following either left or right lesions. Recently Thal and her colleagues (Thal et al., 1991) have studied children with pre- or perinatal left or right lesions, evidencing the early delays in lexical comprehension and naming that these children often present. Similarly we have observed that, during the preschool years, several of the left-lesioned children have been delayed in syntactic development. These initial delays, however, typically lessen over time and by school age, few are considered to present clinically significant deficits requiring language therapy.

In drawing parallels to children with developmental language disorders of unknown origin, it is therefore possible that some such children with delayed language but good outcome by school age may have previously undetected focal lesions, presumably necessitating some degree of reorganisation of language functioning, possibly giving rise to the initial delays in language development. Beyond the early preschool years, these children generally function well, with only subtle deficits remaining.

Depending upon the population served, however, there are a sizeable number of developmental language disordered children who present significantly more marked disorders and for whom prognosis is not as favourable. Among such children are those with significant comprehension disorders, semantic–pragmatic disorders, or developmental verbal apraxia. Except in the acute period following lesion onset, we have never observed such severe forms of language disorders following unilateral lesions in the children with unilateral lesions that we have studied. These more severe forms of language disorders in children have been observed in association with diffuse brain involvement (van Dongen, Loonen and van Dongen, 1985; Van Hout, Evrard and Lyon, 1985; Van Hout and Lyon, 1986). Such observations have led me to conclude that focal lesions generally are not sufficient to result in long-standing, clinically significant forms of language disorders, such as often observed among children with developmental language disorders (Aram, Ekelman and Nation, 1984). Rather, it appears that we have to turn to consideration of more widespread brain involvement to explain many of the developmental forms of developmental language disorders, perhaps at a metabolic or neurotransmitter level and/or perhaps in part genetically transmitted.

## Acknowledgements

Preparation of this manuscript was supported by NIH grant number NS17366.

## References

ALAJOUANINE, T.H. and LHERMITTE, F. (1965). Acquired aphasia in children. *Brain*, **88**(4), 653–662.

ARAM, D.M. and EISELE, J.A. (1991). Plasticity and recovery of higher cortical functions following early brain injury. In: I.Rapin and S.J. Segalowitz (Eds), *Handbook of Neuropsychology: Child Neuropsychology*. New York: Elsevier Science Publishing Co. (In press)

ARAM, D.M. and EKELMAN, B.L. (1987). Unilateral brain lesions in childhood: Performance on the Revised Token Test. *Brain and Language*, **32**, 137–158.

ARAM, D.M. and EKELMAN, B.L. (1988). Auditory temporal perception of children with left or right brain lesions. *Neuropsychologia*, **26**, 931–935.

ARAM, D.M., EKELMAN, B.L. and NATION, J.E. (1984). Preschoolers with language disorders: Ten years later. *Journal of Speech and Hearing Research*, **27**, 232–244.

ARAM, D.M., EKELMAN, B.L. and WHITAKER, H.A. (1986). Spoken syntax in children with acquired unilateral hemisphere lesions. *Brain and Language*, **27**, 75–100.

ARAM, D.M., EKELMAN, B.L. and WHITAKER, H.A. (1987). Lexical retrieval in left and right brain lesioned children. *Brain and Language*, **31**, 61–87.

ARAM, D.M., ROSE, D.F., REKATE, H.L. and WHITAKER, H.A. (1983). Acquired capsular/striatal aphasia in childhood. *Archives of Neurology*, **40**, 614–617.

CARTER, R.L., HOHENEGGER, M.K., and SATZ, P. (1982). Aphasia and speech organization in children. *Science*, **219**, 797–799.

CRANBERG, L.D., FILLEY, C.M., HART, E.J. and ALEXANDER, M.P. (1987). Acquired aphasia in childhood: Clinical and CT investigations. *Neurology*, **37**(7), 1165–1172.

DENCKLA, M.B. and RUDEL, R.G. (1976). Rapid 'automatized' naming (R.A.N.): Dyslexia differentiated from other learning disabilities. *Neuropsychologia*, **14**, 471–479.

DENNIS, M. (1980). Strokes in childhood I: Communicative intent, expression, and comprehension after left hemisphere arteriopathy in a right-handed nine-year old. In: R.W. Rieber (Ed.), *Language Development and Aphasia in Children*, pp. 45–67. New York: Academic Press.

DENNIS, M. and KOHN, B. (1975). Comprehension of syntax in infantile hemiplegics after cerebral hemidecortication: Left hemisphere superiority. *Brain and Language*, **2**, 472–482.

DENNIS, M., LOVETT, M. and WIEGEL-CRUMP, C.A. (1981). Written language acquisition after left or right hemidecortication in infancy. *Brain and Language*, **12**, 54–91.

DENNIS, M. and WHITAKER, H. (1976). Language acquisition following hemidecortication: Linguistic superiority of the left over the right hemisphere. *Brain and Language*, **3**, 404–443.

DE RENZI, E. and VIGNOLO, L.A. (1962). The Token Test: A sensitive test to detect receptive disturbances in aphasics. *Brain*, **85**, 665–678.

EISELE, J. (1991). Selective deficits in language comprehension following early left and right hemisphere damage. In: Martins, I., Castro-Caldas, A., van Dongen, H. and Van Hout, A. (Eds), *Acquired Aphasia in Children*. NATO ASI Series. Dordrecht: Kluwer Academic Publishers.

EISELE, J. and ARAM, D.M. (1992). Differential effects of early hemisphere damage on lexical comprehension and production. *Aphasiology*, in press.

FERRO, J.M., MARTINS, I.P., PINTO, F. and CASTRO-CALDAS, A. (1982). Aphasia following right striato-insular infarction in a left-handed child: A clinico-radiological study. *Developmental Medicine and Child Neurology*, **24**, 173–182.

FLETCHER, J.M. and LEVIN, H.S. (1988). Neurobehavioral effects of brain injury in children. In: D. K. Routh (Ed.), *Handbook of Pediatric Psychology*, pp. 258–295. New York: Guilford Press.

GUTTMANN, E. (1942). Aphasia in children. *Brain*, **65**, 205–219.

HECAEN, H. (1976). Acquired aphasia in children and the ontogenesis of hemispheric functional specialization. *Brain and Language*, **3**, 114–134.

KERSHNER, J.R. and KING, A.J. (1974). Laterality of cognitive functions in achieving hemiplegic children. *Perceptual and Motor Skills*, **39**, 1283–1289.

KIESSLING, L., DENCKLA, M. and CARLTON, M. (1983). Evidence for differential hemispheric function in children with hemiplegic cerebral palsy. *Developmental Medicine and Child Neurology*, **25**, 724–735.

LORING, D.W., MEADOR, K.J., LEE, G.P., MURRO, A.M., SMITH, J.R., FLANIGIN, H.F., GALLAGHER, B.B. and KING, D.W. (1990). Cerebral language lateralization: Evidence from intracarotid amobarbital testing. *Neuropsychologia*, **28**, 831–838.

MARCHMAN, V., MILLER, R. and BATES, E. (1991). Babble and first words in children with focal brain injury. *Applied Psycholinguistics*, **12**, 1–22.

MARTINS, I.P., FERRO, J.M. and TRINDADE, A. (1987). Acquired crossed aphasia in a child. *Developmental Medicine and Child Neurology*, **29**, 96–109.

MCNEIL, M.R. and PRESCOTT, T.E. (1978). *Revised Token Test*. Austin, TX: Pro-Ed, Inc.

MEYERS, S.C., HALL, N.E. and ARAM, D.M. (1990). Fluency and language recovery in a child with a left hemisphere lesion. *Journal of Fluency Disorders*, **15**, 159–173.

PAPANICOLAOU, A.C., DISCENNA, A., GILLESPIE, L.L. and ARAM, D.M. (1990) Probe evoked potential findings following unilateral left hemisphere lesions in children. *Archives of Neurology*, **47**, 562–566.

RANKIN, J.M., ARAM, D.M. and HORWITZ, S.J. (1981). Language ability in right and left hemiplegic children. *Brain and Language*, **12**, 292–306.

RASMUSSEN, T. and MILNER, B. (1977). The role of early left-brain injury in determining lateralization of cerebral speech functions. In: S.J. Dimond and D.A. Blizard (Eds), *Evolution and Lateralization of the Brain. Annals of the New York Academy of Sciences* **299**, 335–369. New York: New York Academy of Sciences.

RIVA, D., CAZZANIGA, L., PANTALEONI, C., MILANI, N. and FEDRIZZI, E. (1986). Acute hemiplegia in childhood: The neuropsychological prognosis. *Journal of Pediatric Neurosciences*, **4**, 239–240.

SHRIBERG, L.D. (1986). *PEPPER: Programs to Examine Phonetic and Phonologic Evaluation Records*. Hillsdale, NJ: Lawrence Erlbaum and Associates.

SHRIBERG, L.D. and ARAM, D.M. (1992) Speech characteristics of brain lesioned children. (Under review.)

SHRIBERG, L.D. and KENT, R.D. (1982). *Clinical Phonetics*. New York: Macmillan.

SHRIBERG, L.D., KWIATKOWSKI, J. and HOFFMANN, K. (1984). A procedure for phonetic transcription by consensus. *Journal of Speech and Hearing Research*, 27, 456–465.

TALLAL, P. (1976). Rapid auditory processing in normal and disordered development. *Journal of Speech and Hearing Disorders*, 30, 3–16.

TALLAL, P. (1987). Developmental language disorders. Report to the U.S. Congress. Interagency Committee on Learning Disabilities, Washington, DC.

TALLAL, P. and NEWCOMBE, F. (1978). Impairment of auditory perception and language comprehension in dysphasia. *Brain and Language*, 5, 13–24.

TALLAL, P. and PIERCY, M. (1973). Developmental aphasia: Impaired rate of non-verbal processing as a function of sensory modality. *Neuropsychologia*, 11, 389–398

TALLAL, P., STARK, R., KALLMAN, C. and MELLITS, D. (1980). Developmental dysphasia: The relation between acoustic processing deficits and verbal processing. *Neuropsychologia*, 18, 273–284.

TALLAL, P., STARK, R. and MELLITS, D. (1985a). The relationship between auditory temporal analysis and receptive language development: Evidence from studies of developmental language disorder. *Neuropsychologia*, 23, 314–322.

TALLAL, P., STARK, R. and MELLITS, D. (1985b). Identification of language-impaired children on the basis of rapid perception and production skills. *Brain and Language*, 25, 314–322.

THAL, D.J., MARCHMAN, V., STILES, J., ARAM, D.M., TRAUNER, D., NASS, R. and BATES, E. (1991). Early lexical development in children with focal brain injury. *Brain and Language*, 40, 491–527

VAN DONGEN, H.R., LOONEN, M.C.B. and VAN DONGEN, K.J. (1985). Anatomical basis for acquired fluent aphasia in children. *Annals of Neurology*, 17, 306–309.

VAN HOUT, A. and LYON, G. (1986). Wernicke's aphasia in a 10-year old boy. *Brain and Language*, 29, 268–285.

VAN HOUT, A., EVRARD, P. AND LYON, G. (1985). On the positive semiology of acquired aphasia in children. *Developmental Medicine and Child Neurology*, 27, 231–241.

VARGHA-KHADEM, F., O'GORMAN, A.M. and WATTERS, G.V. (1985). Aphasia and handedness in relation to hemispheric side, age at injury and severity of cerebral lesion during childhood. *Brain*, 108, 677–696.

VISCH-BRINK, E.G. and SANDT-KOENDERMAN, M. (1984). The occurrence of paraphasias in the spontaneous speech of children with an acquired aphasia. *Brain and Language*, 23, 258–271.

WIEGEL-CRUMP, C.A. and DENNIS, M. (1984). *The Word-Finding Test*. Toronto: The Hospital for Sick Children. (Experimental edition: unpublished test.)

WOODS, B.T. and CAREY, S. (1979). Language deficits after apparent clinical recovery from childhood aphasia. *Annals of Neurology*, 6(5), 405–409.

WOODS, B.T. and TEUBER, H.L. (1978). Changing patterns of childhood aphasia. *Annals of Neurology* 3, 273–280.

# Chapter 7
# Brain imaging
# and language

RICHARD ROBINSON

## Introduction

Enormous efforts have been made over the last 25 years to develop new methods of both structural and functional imaging of the brain. The assumption underlying this effort is that if we can tell where things work (in health) and where things don't work (in sickness), we might be able to learn something about how things work normally. We might even learn about processes of recovery – for example, does recovery depend on relocation of function? This 'localisation' theory was derided as naive almost from when it was first proposed nearly 100 years ago. The controversy has continued with undiminished enthusiasm since. I will attempt to resolve this at the close of this chapter. Meanwhile, whilst on the one hand great insights have been and will continue to be gained into cognitive processes by neuropsychologists who have no interest in brain architecture, a whole generation of clinical neurologists have been profoundly grateful for being able to see on brain images what is wrong with their patients.

## Regional Cortical Blood Flow Imaging

Great interest was aroused in the mid 1970s by a new method of measuring regional cortical blood flow. Brain blood flow is tightly coupled to neuronal metabolism. If neurons become activated they require an immediate increase in delivery of their substrates for energy, glucose and oxygen. Radioactive xenon, $^{133}$Xe, dissolved in blood emits beta rays. Injected into the carotid artery, the beta emissions of separate small areas of brain can be measured and displayed rather in the way a map of the UK is parcelled out into each of the local ordnance survey maps.

Comparing the distribution of blood flow at rest with the altered distribution during some task, one can infer which areas of the brain are working. Thus it was shown (Ingvar and Schwartz, 1974) that hand movement was accompanied by increased flow in the opposite motor and premotor cortex. It is thought that the premotor cortex is where 'programmes' for voluntary movement are 'written' and the motor cortex is the 'hard wiring' from where the preorganised messages are sent to individual muscle groups. If the subject is asked only to think about moving the hand, only the premotor cortex lights up. You can 'see' a thought! Stimulation of the premotor cortex may produce a coordinated movement complex whereas stimulation of the motor cortex produces a single uncoordinated twitch. Similarly an epileptic focus of the premotor cortex will produce complex and often bizarre but involuntary movement sequences whereas an epileptic focus of the motor cortex produces stereotyped recurrent twitching. It is interesting to note how this early observation illuminated not only *how* but *where* motor functions were organised and thereby threw light on not only physiological but also pathological processes. The same group demonstrated that during speech, whilst there was no overall increase in hemisphere flow, there were regional increases in motor and premotor areas involving the vocal apparatus. Abstract thought and mental problem solving increased flow in frontal regions. Further studies (Larsen, Skinhoj and Lessen, 1978) demonstrated that during speech there was a mean (15%) increase in flow in Wernicke's area – implying semantic processing. Interestingly, and at that time unexpectedly, there was a regional increase in right hemisphere flow in similar distribution, but less marked (11%) and more diffuse. Further refinement of the technique has demonstrated that there is a bilateral increase in flow in auditory cortex and its projection areas seen more on the left than the right while listening to words (Nishizawa et al., 1982) but more on the right than on the left were engaged in a task involving analysis of rhythm (Roland, Skinhoj and Lessen, 1981).

The limitations of this technique are that it requires an intracarotid injection, that the occipital lobes supplied by the posterior cerebral arteries are only rather variably demonstrated, that its resolution is limited but above all that it demonstrates changes in blood flow on the brain surface only, not in other important but deeper structures.

## Computed Tomography (CT)

A few years after the start of this functional imaging, CT scanning realised the dream of clinicians to be able to see the brain. Looking back on those early scans which now look as though they were knitted, it is difficult to remember how grateful we were. Its application to patients with aphasia was on the back of an enormous body of knowledge collected painstakingly over many years by linking clinical observation with neuropathological findings after death. The main advantage of CT scanning was that you could be reasonably certain which lesion (in the event of there being more than one) caused which symptoms, and you did not have to wait for your patient to die before attempting to draw clinico-pathological correlations.

The main achievement of work before CT scanning was to classify aphasia into different syndromes in which different symptoms – involving not only language but also motor and perceptual difficulties, clustered together more frequently than might be expected by chance. Although a number of patients could not be fitted neatly into one or other of the increasing number of aphasic syndromes the concept nevertheless held up because a particular language deficit was broadly associated with a particular area of brain damage. In other words this ability to predict within certain limits what part of the brain was affected gave the localisation hypothesis a certain external validity.

Most of the CT correlation was done by collecting a group of patients with similar language problems, i.e. with the same aphasic syndrome, and then analysing the similarity of their CT findings. This was frequently done by standardising the scanning procedures so that the same brain level of each patient was imaged, and then by overlaying the individual images so that it became apparent which brain area they all had in common (Mazzocchi and Vignolo, 1980; Naeser, 1983). This common area was assumed to be the neuropathological core of the syndrome. What emerged was a very smooth transition from neuropathology to CT. For example almost all right-handed aphasics had left-sided lesions.

In order to proceed further a brief description of some of these aphasic syndromes is necessary. The original description by Broca in 1861 of a non-fluent aphasia initiated the history of aphasia. Speech is effortful and limited and perhaps because of this paraphasias are uncommon. Speech repetition is impaired. Writing is similarly disturbed. By contrast, comprehension of the spoken and written word is relatively intact. This might be conceptualised as a disorder between the phonological output lexicon and the response buffer. The most consistent neuropathological substrate for Broca's aphasia is the lower one-third of the left inferior frontal gyrus – sometimes called the frontal operculum or eponymously Broca's area (Mohr et al., 1978; but see Mori, Yamadori and Furumoto 1989).

In 1874 Wernicke described a second condition of language difficulty in some respects the converse of Broca's aphasia. In this syndrome, utterance is fluent with reasonably preserved syntax – although it may be variably deficient in meaning. By contrast, comprehension of the spoken word is severely impaired. There would appear again on neuropsychological models to be a disconnection between the auditory input lexicon and the cognitive system. Experts differ as to precisely which area is involved in these patients but agree that the posterior one-third of the superior temporal gyrus is always affected with a variable involvement ofadjacent cortex posteriorly (Kertesz, 1983). Thus an anterior (motor) to posterior (sensory) spectrum of aphasia began to emerge. Next it was confirmed that patients with global aphasia with severe comprehension *and* speech difficulty had large lesions involving both Broca's and Wernicke's areas.

In time other less common syndromes were described. *Conduction aphasia* is characterised by speech which, although relatively fluent, has word-finding difficulty and phonemic paraphasias. Comprehension is relatively preserved. The hallmark of this syndrome is impaired repetition due, it was hypothesised, to a disconnection between sensory input and motor output systems. CT findings seemed to bear this out with lesions deep to Wernicke's area either in the arcuate fasciculus which connects to the parietal with frontal cortex, or in the white matter deep to the insula which is midway between the two (Benson et al., 1973; Damasio and Damasio, 1983).

In *transcortical sensory aphasia* there appears to be difficulty in transferring from the auditory input lexicon to the cognitive system, hence comprehension is impaired. Here the lesion is usually in the temporooccipital cortex (Kertesz, Sheppard and MacKenzie, 1982). In transcortical motor aphasia the problems may be seen as lying between the cognitive system and phonological output lexicon. Here of course spontaneous speech is impaired and the lesion is in the supplementary motor area of the dominant frontal lobe (Alexander and Schmitt, 1980; Rubens and Kertesz, 1983). The hallmark of these transcortical aphasias is preserved repetition – suggesting that the indirect route from auditory input to phonological output lexicons remains intact.

Finally, increasing numbers of patients with *subcortical aphasias* with a variety of language problems were described (e.g. Basso, della Salla and Farabola, 1987). The lesions were either in the basal ganglia, caudate and putamen, or in the thalamus. It was suggested that a role for the thalamus was to activate cortical areas and that in thalamic damage those areas structurally intact were functionally deactivated.

During this period another isotopic method became available, but this time involving imaging of the whole brain, not just the cortical surface. The findings using radioactive technecium corroborated the CT data but without the architectural detail (Kertesz, Lesk and McCabe, 1977; Soh et al., 1978).

Thus to summarise it appeared that verbal input to the posterior part of the left superior temporal gyrus was processed onwards for phonetic and semantic analysis in the temporoparietal areas. Ouput from this area might consist of conversion of thoughts into words commensurate with their underlying meaning. This neural word representation is projected to the frontal operculum via association fibres for phonological output conversion. From here projection via the supplementary area to the motor cortex served speech output. I have for the sake of brevity not described the relatively secure pathological foundation of pure word deafness at one end of this process or aphemia at the other end.

This scheme of things had its detractors. It was pointed out that the conclusions were based on a population consisting almost entirely of right-handed unilingual white adults speaking an atonal language who wrote in an alphabetic code – conditions applying to less than one-quarter of the human population (Basso et al., 1985). It was argued that lesions could impair function in any one of at least three ways – by destroying functional cortex, by destroying connections to or from the cortex or by inactivating the cortex by damage to more remote structures. It is difficult to tell in individual cases which of these predominates. It was shown that not only did a substantial proportion of patients not fit neatly into one of the described syndromes but also that clinicopathological exceptions were not uncommon. Thus, for example in one series of 207 aphasics with cortical lesions, 36 had unexpected findings (Basso et al., 1985). In another study of patients with global aphasia only 53% had the classical anterior, posterior lesion (Scarpa et al., 1987). The possibility was raised that the syndrome of Broca's aphasia could include a number of language difficulties embracing morphological impairments, syntactic problems, phonological output processing and when analysed carefully even a failure of comprehension of sentence structure information.

Most lesion localisation analysis was carried out on patients who had sustained arterial infarcts frequently including rather similar and large volumes of brain. It might be, particularly when groups of patients rather than individuals were studied, that interesting structural and functional relationships became obscured. All that remained might be a group of language problems joined not by cognitive processes but by an arbitrary, and for these purposes irrelevant, blood supply (Ellis and Young, 1988).

## Positron Emission Tomography (PET)

It is therefore with this slightly shaky neurological framework that we have entered the latest area of functional imaging – PET – whereby not only regional cerebral blood flow but actual cellular metabolism can be imaged by displaying rates of oxygen or glucose uptake. As with the early xenon cortical blood flow studies activated states such as listening, speaking or reading can be compared with resting states. The PET studies may be divided into those physiological studies exploring normal language processing on the one hand and pathological studies documenting changes in aphasia on the other. The former obviously serve to interpret the latter.

Thus monoaural (either left or right) verbal stimuli produce bilateral activation of posterior temporal gyri together with diffuse activation of the left hemisphere. Analysis of monoaural chords again produces bilateral activation but right greater than left frontotemporal asymmetries. Analysis of tone sequence pairs in which the subject is invited to decide whether they are the same or different has been shown to produce differing results depending on whether they are analysed by musically sophisticated listeners (in which case there is left greater than right temporal asymmetry) or by musically naive listeners (right greater than left frontotemporal asymmetry) (Mazziotta et al., 1982).

Sequential studies of changes in cerebral blood flow compared the passive listening state with subjects listening to and then repeating words, thereby distinguishing that component due to output coding and motor control (Peterson et al., 1988). Comparing the blood flow changes occurring on repetition of heard words with blood flow changes occurring when subjects were asked to associate a use for each word (e.g. for 'cake – eat') distinguished areas involved in semantic processing.

It comes as no surprise that passive listening increased activity in superior temporal areas (left more than right) and that with speech the supplementary motor area and primary motor cortex for lips and mouth were involved. When semantic processing was undertaken, the inferior anterior frontal cortex, left greatly in excess of right was involved. This is a new finding which implies a needed re-evaluation of the involvement of the frontal lobe anterior to Broca's area in language processing.

Early PET studies in aphasic patients also threw up interesting results supporting some of the criticisms of CT lesional data. Their cerebral metabolism is almost invariably depressed in areas larger than and at times remote from the lesion apparent on CT scans, implying disconnection or de-activation. Thus a patient with a clinical picture consistent with thalamic aphasia (anomia and perseveration with spared repetition and comprehension) with an intact thalamus on CT scanning showed depressed metabolism not only in the left thalamus but also in the left middle and inferior temporal gyri (Metter et al., 1981). Almost invariably thalamic involvement is present in aphasia. This, however, is a non-specific finding – also present in strokes without aphasia when the thalamus itself is damaged – implying secondary de-activation of structural intact cortex, the decrease in thalamic blood flow or metabolism is greater than when the thalamus is secondarily involved due to damaged cortex. Further studies (Metter et al., 1988) have supported the role of subcortical structures having major effects on frontal lobe metabolism.

Larger functional depression than lesions apparent to CT scan appears to be the rule with patients with Broca's aphasia where commonly the entire left hemisphere (with the exception of the primary visual cortex) is seen to be involved on PET imaging. In Wernicke's aphasia not only is there the expected temporoparietal involvement but also moderate reduction in prefrontal activity. It has been suggested that this is the result of lack of input from temporoparietal cortex. The impulse to speech is not impeded but this lack of semantic input results in failure to monitor what is said. Similarly, in conduction aphasia wider areas of involvement necessary than for strict disconnection between Broca's and Wernicke's area appear to be the rule (Kempler et al., 1988). It should be noted at this point that activation studies in aphasia, for example listening to speech or attempting to speak, have yet to be published.

This is for the very good reason that everybody is rethinking the neurophysiology of language, not in terms of the strict one-to-one site-to-function relationship in the way I earlier described but in terms of functionally overlapping networks. There may be a bias towards a particular aspect of function at a particular locus but it is by no means exclusive. There are extensive interconnections not only between particular language sites but also between language sites and areas concerned with uni- and multimodal perceptual processing. The meaning of the word is likely to be represented by a network which includes not only neurones concerned with perceptual processing but also networks involving memory, as well as other limbic structures entraining an affective component.

These considerations explain why in PET language activation studies many areas are activated apparently simultaneously. It is not surprising therefore that careful analysis of language function in non-fluent aphasics with damage in Broca's area reveals difficulty in understanding sentences when their meaning is influenced by preposition and word order. Silent generation of single words without syntactical connotations causes activation of Broca's area and supplementary motor area. This is rather like the equivalent of thinking of moving the arm referred to earlier. It appears impossible to separate the semantics of a word from its motor representation. Stimulation of Broca's area may block phoneme identification implying some role in auditory analysis. Conversely, stimulation of Wernicke's area can interfere with coordination of pharyngeal movement causing speech arrest – although not as consistently as with stimulation of Broca's areas.

The sensory/motor divide is increasingly seen as being relative rather than absolute. The major language 'centres' may represent a convergence of a number of parallel networks each with a varying bias towards a particular type of language function. Aphasia thus becomes a restraint on information processing rather than an absolute block in a language pathway.

## The Right Hemisphere

We have seen from all the cerebral blood flow and regional metabolic studies that there is bihemispheric involvement in language. This has largely been ignored by clinical neurologists since right hemisphere damage rarely leads to aphasia. The neuropsychological community have shown more enterprise. Speech following right hemisphere damage tends to be excessive and rambling with irrelevant comments often focusing on insignificant details; thus in retelling stories there is difficulty in drawing proper inferences. Careful testing reveals an insensitivity to the pragmatic elements of discourse. Thus there is an inability fully to appreciate other speaker's intentions, the purpose of conversational exchange or listener's needs. Further, there are difficulties with complex non-contexted bound language such as jokes and metaphors (Caramazza et al., 1976). For example, 'face the music' may be given a literal rather than a figurative interpretation. There is difficulty in selecting the appropriate punch line to end a joke. A further difficulty is in identifying affective intonation, particularly if the posterior right hemisphere is affected. Anterior right hemisphere damage tends to lead to monotonous speech. Here we have an echo of the left hemisphere anterior (motor)–posterior (sensory) spectrum. Thus it would seem that the right hemisphere explores metaphorical aspects between words and word association where the left hemisphere processes alternative word meanings. For a full richness of all semantic aspects integration between the two hemispheres is necessary.

## Childhood Aphasia

Most of this account has been based on studies in adults. Studies on acquired aphasia in children tend to emphasise their comparatively good recoverability. This has been ascribed to the facility of children for transferring language function from the left to the right hemisphere. From studies involving intracarotid injection of sodium amytal, briefly anaesthetising one hemisphere, it appears that children who acquire the aphasic insult before the age of 6 years are more likely to acquire right hemisphere 'dominance' for language than if the insult is acquired later (Milner, 1974). However, perhaps we should now appreciate that terms such as language 'dominance' are less appropriate to this situation.

What we should be looking for in children with early acquired aphasia is an attempted meshing of all aspects of language function in the same hemisphere. Recovery from childhood aphasia is not always as complete as it might seem. It would be interesting to know to what extent this might be attributed to an incomplete meshing process. It would also be of interest to look at the child's and adult's ability to transfer right hemispheric language function to the left hemisphere following right hemisphere damage.

## Developmental Language Disorders

A further issue is to what extent do the, albeit tentative, conclusions from aphasia apply to developmental language problems. One small study (Lou, Henrixsen and Bruhn, 1990), using a technique similar to PET, suggested that four children with a lexical/semantic deficit had blood flow lower in the left central perisylvian region than the right, whereas three children with phonological/syntactic problems had left prefrontal flow lower than the right. This limited information is at least congruent with studies of postnatally acquired pathology. Little is known of the neuropathology of developmental language disorders. One temporoparietal structure, the planum temporale, has long been known to be normally larger on the left than the right (from birth), a fact traditionally associated with left hemisphere language 'dominance'. Morphometric analysis of the planum temporale in dyslexic children suggests this structure is symmetrical or even has reversed asymmetry (right larger than left) (Hynd and Semrud-Cliheman, 1989). I would, however, sound a note of caution here about detailed morphological studies based on non-invasive imaging. No two individual gyral patterns are precisely the same, but more importantly the functional and microscopically distinct boundaries do not correspond to gyral architecture. Perhaps more significant therefore is the pathological evidence for failure of completely organised neuronal migration in dyslexia (Hynd and Semrud-Cliheman, 1989). This implies a failure of neuronal organisation early in fetal life. It is difficult to see, even with our most advanced imaging techniques, how we would be able to detect and study changes at this morphological level. I would suggest that individual case studies with comprehensive analysis of both right and left language hemisphere function in individuals with small circumscribed lesions (identified metabolically rather than architecturally) might be a more rewarding approach.

## Conclusions

There is no doubt that localisation has been essential for the study of brain function in the non-human primate and other animal models. From these studies much that is valuable for an understanding about perceptual processing movement and memory function in the human has been achieved. For obvious reasons the same method cannot he applied to the study of language. A complete description of the brain must involve both structure and function. Even our broad-brush approximation of the two in the area of language has done much to help people with neurological disease. Ideas about structure have moved away from localities with clear cut boundaries to the foci of multiple networks. I believe that the reward will be correspondingly great as we attempt finer grain detail whilst keeping both aspects of the brain in view.

## References

ALEXANDER, M. P. and SCHMITT M.A. (1980). The aphasia syndrome of stroke in the left anterior artery territory. *Archives of Neurology*, 37, 97–100

BASSO, A. DELLA SALLA, S. and FARABOLA, M. (1987). Aphasia arising from purely deep lesions. *Cortex*, 23, 29–44.

BASSO, A. LECOURS, A.R., MORASCHINI, S. and VAINER, M. (1985).Anatomicoclinical correlations of the aphasia as defined through computerised tomography: exceptions. *Brain and Language*, 26, 201–229.

BENSON, D.F., SHEREMATE, W.A., BOUCHARD, R., SEGARRA, S.M., PRICE, D. and GESCHWIND, N. (1973). Conduction aphasia: a clinicopathological study. *Archives of Neurology*, 28, 339–346.

CARAMAZZA, A., GOBDON, J., ZURIF, E.B. and DE LUCA, D. (1976). Right hemispheric damage and verbal problem solving behaviour. *Brain and Language*, 6, 41–46.

DAMASIO, H. and DAMASIO, A.R. (1983). Localisation of lesions in conduction aphasia. In: Kertesz, A. (Ed), *Localisation in Neuropsychology*. London, New York: Academic Press.

ELLIS, A.N. and YOUNG, A.W. (1988). *Human Cognitive Neuropsychology*. Hillsdale, N.J.: Lawrence Erlbaum and Associates.

HYND, G. W. AND SEMRUD-CLIHEMAN, M.(1989). Dyslexia and brain morphology. *Psychological Bulletin*, 106, 447–482.

INGVAR, D.H. and SCHWARTZ, M. (1974). Blood flow patterns in the dominant hemisphere by speech and reading. *Brain*, 97, 273–288.

KEMPLER, D. METTER, J. JACKSON, C.A. HANSON, W.R. RIEGE, W.H. MAZZIOTTA, J.and PHELPS, M.E. (1988). Disconnection and cerebral metabolism. The case of conduction aphasia. *Archives of Neurology*, 45, 275–279.

KERTESZ, A. (Ed.) (1983). Localisation of lesions in Wernicke's aphasia. In: Kertesz, A. (Ed.) *Localisation in Neuropsychology*. London, New York: Academic Press.

KERTESZ, A., LESK, A. and MCCABE, P. (1977). Isotope localisation of infarcts in aphasia. *Archives of Neurology*, 34, 590–601.

KERTESZ, A. SHEPPARD, A. and MACKENZIE, R. (1982). Localisation in trans-cortical sensory aphasia. *Archives of Neurology*, 39, 475–478.

LARSEN, B. SKINHOJ, E. and LESSEN, N.A. (1978). Variation in regional cortical blood flow in the right and left hemisphere during automatic speech. *Brain*, 101, 193–211.

LOU, H.C., HENRIXSEN, L. and BRUHN, P. (1990). Focal cerebral dysfunction in developmental learning disabilities. *Lancet*, 8–11.

MAZZIOTTA, J.C., PHELPS, N.E., CARSON, R.E. & KUHL, D.E. (1982). Thermographic mapping of the auditory cortex during auditory stimulation. *Neurology*, 32, 921–937.

MAZZOCCHI, F. and VIGNOLO, L. (1980). Localisation of lesions in aphasia: clinical CT correlation in stroke patients. *Cortex*, 15, 627–654.

METTER, E.J., RIEGE, E., HANSON, W.R., JACKSON, C.A., KEMPLER, D. and VAN LANCHER, D. (1988). Sub-cortical structures in aphasia: an analysis based on (F-18) Fluorodeoxyglucose Positron Emission Tomography and Computed Tomography. *Archives of Neurology*, 45, 1229–1234.

METTER, E.J., WASTERLAIN, C.G., KUHL, D.E., HANSON, W. and PHELPS, N.E., (1981). FGD Positron Emission Computed Tomography in the study of aphasia. *Annals of Neurology*, 10, 173–183.

MILNER, B. (1974). Hemispheric Specialisation: Scope and limits. In: Schmitt, F.O. and Worden, F. J. (Eds), *The Neurosciences Third Study Programme*. Cambridge, MA: MIT Press.

MOHR, J.P., PESSIN, M.S., FINKELSTEIN, S., FINKELSTEIN, H.H. DUNCAN, T.W. and DAVIS, K.R. (1978). Broca Aphasia: pathological and clinical. *Neurology*, 28, 311–324.

MORI, E., YAMADORI, A. and FURUMOTO, M. (1989). Left pre-central girus and Broca's Aphasia: a clinicopathological study. *Neurology*, 39, 51–57.

NAESER, M.A. (1983). CT Scan lesion size and lesion locus in cortical and sub-cortical aphasias. In: Kertesz, A. (Ed.), *Localisation and Neuropsychology*. London, New York: Academic Press.

NISHIZAWA, Y., OLSEN, T.S., LARSEN, B. and LASSEN, N.A. (1982) Left–right cortical asymmetries of regional cerebral blood flow during listening to words. *Journal of Neurophysiology*, 48, 458–466.

PETERSON, S.C., FOX, B.T., POSNER, M.I., MINTUN, M. and RAICHLE, M. (1988). PET studies of the cortical anatomy of single word processing. *Nature*, 331, 585–589.

ROLAND, P.E., SKLNHOJ, E. and LASSEN, N.A. (1981). Focal activation of human cerebral cortex during auditory discrimination. *Journal of Neurophysiology*, 45, 1139–1151.

RUBENS, A.B. and KERTESZ, A. (1983). The localisation of lesions in transcortical aphasia. In: Kertesz, A. (Ed.), *Localisation in Neuropsychology*. London, New York: Academic Press.

SCARPA, M., COLOMBO, A., SORGATO, P. and DE RENZI, E. (1987). The incidence of aphasia and global aphasia in left brain damaged patients. *Cortex*, 23, 331–336.

SOH, LARSEN, B. SKINHOJ, E. and LESSEN, N.A. (1978). Regional cerebral blood flow in aphasia. *Archives of Neurology*, 35, 625–632.

# Chapter 8
# Cognitive abilities of language-impaired children

JUDITH R. JOHNSTON

I began my studies of language disorder as a clinician. Even now, when I think of 'specific language impairment', I think of the children:

- Mark, a four year old at the two-word stage, assuming the role of his mother in a complicated pretend-play drama set at the movie theatre.
- Lisa, a six year old at the one-word stage, laughing at her own puns.
- Alex, a four year old with no expressive speech, showing other children in our preschool how to make vegetable tempura.

Children with specific language impairment are, by definition, children for whom the development of language and thought is out of phase. Each of my illustrative children had knowledge and competencies far in advance of what you would expect from their language levels. Each of them had achieved normal-range scores on a non-verbal test of intelligence. Each of them, at times, radiated a fierce intellectual energy that was undeniable. In short, they seemed like classic examples of children who are intellectually normal though language delayed. The problem is this: by virtually any account of intellect, such children should not exist.

## Developmental Relationships Between Cognition and Language

To understand why this is so, we need to consider the many relationships between language and thought, or to be more precise, between verbal and non-verbal cognition. Studying patterns of human growth, we quickly discover that the development of language and thought are interdependent, at all stages of life. Consider first the relationship between cognition and language which is evident in the learning of language. The nature of this process is controversial, but I am among those who hold that the 'language acquisition device' is nothing more or less than the general information-processing capabilities that constitute the mind itself. From this perspective, children learn the language system by applying their powers of observation, organisation and analysis to the examples of language that they hear. Awesome as these powers may be, cognitive scientists have long argued that the mind functions as a limited capacity system, that is, as a system that can only do so much at once. In complex tasks, this restriction may lead to processing 'tradeoffs' . For example, most drivers can converse while driving – until the traffic gets heavy. Similar phenomena can be seen in young language learners. Toddlers are more likely to use new inflectional morphemes when expressing familiar semantic relations (Leonard, Steckol and Schwartz, 1978). Utterances with greater propositional complexity are less likely to include all of the underlying constituents (Bloom, Miller and Hood, 1975). And young children's syntactic errors increase with syllabic complexity (Panagos and Prelock, 1982). The notion of limited capacity seems quite applicable to these examples. Other principles of mental function, e.g. recency and interruption effects in memory, or attentional biases towards novelty, could likewise be shown to influence language learning and use (e.g. Pinker, 1989). The most fundamental relationship between cognition and language, then, is that cognitive mechanisms create, and constrain, language knowledge.

Different relationships between cognition and language are evident when we look before and after the language learning phase. Before they can learn to speak, infants must learn to think about means and ends, and to understand the limits imposed by the independence of objects (Bates et al., 1979). These non-verbal, cognitive achievements help prepare toddlers to use words as symbolic tools of communication. Once language is learned, however, the dependencies shift. Language becomes a major mode of mental representation and crucial to many reasoning tasks. Depictive imagery may suffice when one's goal is to rearrange the living room, but other goals require the unique power of words to represent just those aspects of objects and events that are pertinent to the problem. Consider the business manager preparing a work assignment plan, or a teenager choosing between two summer jobs. It is hard to imagine success in such tasks without the use of language. Words are a powerful and flexible way to create non-existent events for reflection and organising (Olson, 1975).

To summarise briefly, language is normally a well-integrated part of mental life. We apply the organising forces of non-verbal intellect to learn language in the first place, and we rely constantly on language symbols for complex reasoning. Language would seem to be both the product and the tool of cognition. If so, children with specific language impairment should not exist. If language is late and slow to develop, there should be a cognitive reason. If language symbols are poorly controlled, there should be a cognitive consequence.

## Studies of Cognitive Development in Children with Specific Language Impairment

### Symbolic Play

About 12 years ago, I, my students and other investigators began to look more carefully at the putative normal intellect of children with specific language impairment. Let me summarise briefly what we have found. One group of studies has examined symbolic play in this population. A report by Terrell et al. (1984) will illustrate this line of research. Fifteen normal and 15 language-impaired children were asked to complete the Symbolic Play Test (Lowe and Costello, 1976) and to engage in spontaneous pretend play activities. The children were all at the one-word stage and had expressive vocabularies of 25–75 words; the language-impaired group was a year and a half older than the normal group, i.e. 35 months versus 19 months. Play samples were rated according to such properties as the number of symbolic acts, the number of play units combining two or more symbolic schemes, and the number of play units which focused on actors other than the self. The language-impaired children engaged in more complex and mature play than their language peers, but they fell significantly below age expectations. Similar findings have been reported in at least eight other investigations (Lovell, Hoyle and Siddall, 1968; Morehead, 1972; Brown et al., 1975; Udwin and Yule, 1983; Roth and Clark, 1987; Skarakis and Prutting, 1988; Terrell and Schwartz, 1988; Thal and Bates, 1988).

### Conceptual Development

A second group of studies has used Piagetian paradigms to assess conceptual development in children with specific language impairment (Snyder, 1978; Camarata, Newhoff and Rugg, 1981; Kamhi, 1981; Siegel et al., 1981; Johnston and Ramstad, 1983; Camarata, Newhoff and Rugg, 1985). Kamhi's work (1981) can be taken as representative of the set. In his study, a group of five-year-old children with specific language impairment was compared with two normal groups, one matched to the impaired group by mental age, the other by language level. Each of the children was given six reasoning tasks, ranged across the conceptual domains of space, class, and number. As parts of this battery, children had to sort geometric shapes which varied in size, colour and shape; arrange small toys in order, according to a visible model; determine the relative quantity of two sets of checkers; and recognise geometric shapes by feel. Each of these tasks has a long research history and provides a reliable picture of the maturity of a child's thought. In this light, Kamhi's findings are particularly telling: in each of the six tasks, the language-impaired children out-performed their language peers, but failed to reach the performance level of their mental age peers. Not many of the individual comparisons were statistically significant, but the likelihood of obtaining this consistent pattern of results by chance alone is virtually nil. Moreover, these results are in general accord with those from other studies, including ones that have observed older children (Johnston and Ramstad, 1983), and ones that have used strictly non-verbal adaptations of the Piagetian tasks (Siegel, et al., 1981).

*Summary of Data*

There have been other efforts to study cognitive development in children with language impairment, but these two bodies of research will serve to provide an initial answer to our question. (See Johnston, 1988, and Bishop, 1991, for comprehensive reviews.) We have seen how theories of the relationship between cognition and language predict that children with specific language impairment should not exist. The reports of symbolic play and conceptual development indicate that, indeed, they don't – at least not in the classic sense. When we observe children who have normal non-verbal IQs and serious language delays, they in fact seem to be lacking the conceptual knowledge, the representational abilities, and the reasoning patterns that would be expected for their age.

## The Nature of the Cognitive Disability

*The Role of Language in Cognitive Impairment*

Should we believe these data? Could they merely be reflections of the language disorder itself? Experimenters can minimise the demands for explicit language use, but that scarcely prevents children from using language as an internal mental tool. Perhaps the language-impaired children performed less well than their age peers merely because they lack facility with such inner speech? Note that this line of argument implies that some mental calculations welcome verbal representation even if they don't require it. Non-verbal strategies for such problems might exist in principle but prove clumsy or complex in application, leading to breakdowns in reasoning or delayed mastery. By this scenario, whenever verbal strategies lead to simpler solutions than non-verbal strategies, the child with a language impairment would be at a developmental disadvantage. Language would be crucial for solving these problems at a given age or stage, if not absolutely. My first answer to the skeptic is thus: yes, poor performance on symbolic or conceptual tasks could indeed reflect a lack of facility with the inner use of language. However, that is not a problem for these data, that is their point.

*Evidence for Non-verbal Deficits*

What the skeptic really wants to know, of course, is whether there is any evidence to indicate that the cognitive deficits of language-impaired children extend to non-verbal functions. Difficulties with rhythm perception (Kracke, 1975), and memory for spatial arrays (Doehring, 1960; Wyke and Asso, 1979) would seem to suggest purely non-verbal impairments. The most convincing data on this point, however, may come from an imagery study conducted by Ellis Weismer and myself. We asked language impaired and normal children at 6;6 and 9;6 years of age to judge whether or not two rows of geometric forms were the same. They pressed a response panel to indicate their answer. In one-quarter of the items, both arrays were presented in vertical orientation. In the remaining items, the right-hand array was rotated about its centre 45, 90 or 135 degrees. All of the children were screened for their understanding of spatial order concepts and were trained with the apparatus, with emphasis on both accuracy and speed. The ultimate variable for group comparison was response time.

An important feature of this paradigm is that patterns of response across the items can reveal the nature of the mental strategy that was used to solve the problem (Kosslyn, 1980). If the viewer solves the problem by creating and manipulating mental images, response time proves to be a direct function of the degree of rotation. Extended rotations require more time. If the viewer solves the problem by using verbal symbols to represent the two arrays, the relationship between response time and degree of rotation does not hold. This fact about the task paradigm makes the results of our study particularly interesting. First, data patterns clearly showed that the language-impaired children were using non-verbal, imagistic strategies. Second, although the language-impaired children were accurate in their judgements of order, their response times were substantially slower than those of the control group. This difference remained true even after we adjusted response times to control for any speed differences that were evident during training. Faced with changing arrays, language-impaired children took longer to make judgements of spatial order. Taken together, these findings indicate that the cognitive deficits of language impaired children do extend to non-verbal functions.

*The Inadequacy of Current Proposals*

There remains little room for doubt on the original question. Across a range of tasks and ages, children with specific language impairment have shown a marked level of intellectual impairment. A portion of this cognitive disability must reflect the role of language in higher level problem solving. Without normal verbal facility, the language-impaired child is unlikely to reach normal levels of achievement on tasks which require the consideration of multiple hypothetical states. Another portion of the cognitive disability is non-verbal and can be presumed to be responsible for inefficient learning in many domains, including language. Here many questions remain, not the least of which concern the fundamental nature of the problem. Some investigators have proposed that language-impaired children have difficulty with particular complex mental activities such as hierarchical planning (Cromer, 1983), symbolic function (Morehead, 1972), or hypothesis testing (Nelson, Kamhi and Apel, 1987). Others have proposed difficulty with basic mechanisms of auditory perception (Eisenson, 1968), attention (Mackworth, Grandstaff and Pribram, 1973; Ceci, 1983) or short-term memory (Kirchner and Klatzky, 1985). Ultimately, none of these proposals fit the data.

*Illustrative Data and Interpretation: Capacity Limitations.* One of my own studies, with its explanatory arguments, will serve to illustrate the troubled state of current theorising. Johnston and Smith (1988) observed preschool children with and without language impairment as they solved a series of complex communication problems. On each item, the children were shown three objects varying systematically in size, colour and identity. In the dimensional sets, two of the objects were similar on the target dimension, e.g. colour, but differed on the second dimension, e.g. size; the third object differed from the first two in the target dimension, but resembled one of them on the second dimension. For example, one object set might consist of a large green peg, a small green peg and a large purple peg. In the identity sets, two of the objects were identical while the third differed from the first two in every respect. As each item began, the examiner would point to two, similar, objects from the set of three. The child's task was to describe these objects to a puppet so that the puppet would know which ones to take.

All of the children were successful in the referential task, providing communicatively adequate descriptions. However, the language-impaired children used descriptive strategies which were characteristically different from those provided by their peers. Across all items, responses fell into six categories, illustrated here for an item in which two green pegs are the designated referents:

| | |
|---|---|
| *1. Deictic* | 'This one and that one' |
| *2. Exhaustive* | 'A green big one and a green little one' |
| *3. Exclusive* | 'Not the purple one' |
| *4. Iterative* | 'The green one and the green one' |
| *5. Partitive* | 'Looks like little and green big' |
| *6. Quantitative grouping* | 'Two green ones' |

Note that all of these strategies, except no.1, require dimensional analysis. Strategy 6 additionally requires that the two targeted objects be considered as a quantified set. The key finding was this: language-impaired children used the Quantitative Grouping strategy much less often than their normal peers when describing objects that were similar in size or colour. Performance on the identity items was not so restricted. When they did not need to consider separate dimensions, the language impaired children frequently described objects with phrases such as 'the two house' . They also demonstrated knowledge of all the requisite dimensional terms. In short, their problem seemed to stem, not from a lack of knowledge schemes, but from some inability to make use of these schemes to solve a particular problem. To quote from our original report, 'Given a task which welcomed the combined use of two higher-level, complex processing routines, the impaired children used one or the other more often than both. The data thus seem to represent the variable performance of thinkers who are operating near the limits of their processing resources.'

*Critique of Capacity Limitation as an Explanation of Cognitive Disability.* How viable is this suggestion that language-impaired children suffer limitations in processing capacity? Like other appeals to basic cognitive mechanisms, this explanation has the advantage of being content free and thus applicable to diverse mental tasks. It differs in this regard from explanations which focus on particular sorts of mental activities such as symbol use or hierarchical structuring. The notion of capacity limitations also applies equally well across perceptual modalities, and to both verbal and non-verbal functions. It thus fits the growing body of data that indicates visual as well as auditory perceptual disorders (Tallal, 1990), and non-verbal as well as verbally mediated deficits. Finally, the notion of capacity limitations would predict both the observed delays in concept/scheme attainment and the observed failures in concept/scheme deployment. Each mental calculation enhances control of available schemes and brings the opportunity for new discoveries. Processing limitations could easily hamper both sorts of mental growth. In sum, explanations of cognitive deficit based on notions of limitations in processing capacity have particular appeal because they seem to fit the broad range of performance data.

As is frequently the case, the broad scope of this explanation may prove to be its Achilles heel. Global appeals to capacity limitation are difficult to reconcile with evidence of selective impairment, and such evidence definitely exists. Children with specific language impairments do complete the tasks on non-verbal intelligence scales with normal proficiency. They do perform better on non-verbal tasks than on verbal tasks (e.g. Kamhi, 1981; Terrell et al., 1984), and, in the world of language, they do seem to learn words faster than they do grammatical morphemes (Moore, 1990). Any explanation of cognitive impairment must also account for these instances of selective sparing. Arguments about capacity limitations must thus be accompanied by detailed analyses which show why a processing mechanism flawed in this fashion succeeds better on some tasks than on others. For example, in our recent study of dimensional reasoning (Johnston and Smith, 1988), we argue that inferences about size demand more processing resources than inferences about colour because size judgements are inherently ordinal and colour judgements are not. Explanations of this sort will be more difficult to construct across varying task paradigms and developmental levels, but without them, arguments about capacity limitations will remain quite hollow. We might begin this analytic work by compiling a list of the task parameters which have seemed to account for differential performance. Siegel et al. (1981) note that the more difficult tasks in their battery required 'sequential processing'. Kamhi (1981) suggests that his difficult tasks required 'anticipatory images'. Inhelder (1976) implies that the more difficult tasks will be ones that cannot be solved with 'schemes of actual physical action.' Clahsen (1989) concludes that grammatical morphemes are relatively difficult because of the 'scope' of the rules that govern them. If we can translate these, and other similar, ideas into the language of processing complexity, we may be able to explain how a pervasive impairment can lead to selective performance deficits.

Even if we succeed in this task, however, we face two further problems with the notion of capacity limitation. The first is that some of the evidence of cognitive deficit in language-impaired children comes from tasks which cannot be construed as complex. The reports of Tallal and her colleagues provide the clearest examples (e.g. Tallal and Piercy, 1973; Tallal et al., 1981). In these experiments, children perform perceptual discrimination tasks such as identifying the order of two tones that are presented with various silent intervals between them. The language-impaired children have extreme difficulty with the shortest intervals, but perform as well as their peers with the longer intervals. These findings clearly imply a processing deficit, but not one that is obviously related to capacity limitations. Rather, as Tallal (1988) concludes, 'children with specific developmental language disorders, as a group, are characterized by an inability to perceive and to produce information rapidly in time.' At the very least it would seem that cognitive processing explanations of intellectual impairment will need to invoke limitations in rate as well as capacity. Or will they?

This question is prompted by one final problem with the notion of capacity limitation. In many recent models of cognition, capacity is treated as a matter of function, not structure (Kail and Bisanz, 1982; Chi and Gallagher, 1982). Thus construed, capacity is tantamount to workload, or accomplishment, within a given unit of time. Work that is more rapid, more efficient and/or done with more powerful mental schemes, can lead to increased capacity. On the other hand, slower rates of processing, less efficient access to information, or the need to use more schemes of narrow scope can lead to capacity limitations. In such a system, 'capacity' is the epiphenomenal product of an interaction of variables such as rate, efficiency and power. Capacity may be the construct that we know how best to measure, but it fails as a satisfying explanation. We may need to learn from the experience of those cognitive scientists who have abandoned their research on this construct altogether (Allport, 1989).

## Research Achievements and Challenges

It is time now to summarise my main line of argument. The developmental relationships between cognition and language make it unlikely that a child could be seriously delayed in language acquisition and otherwise normal in intellect. Research over the past decade has revealed that children with specific language impairment do, in fact, show cognitive delays and deficits across a considerable range of tasks. The challenge for researchers now is to determine the nature of the cognitive disorder which underlies these observations. Those of us who work within the frameworks of cognitive science have been attracted by the explanatory potential of constructs like capacity limitation, but we are also discovering the complexity of applying these notions to the performance profiles of children with specific language impairment. I suspect that those pursuing other hypotheses will discover analogous problems.

Despite a temporary plateau in our studies of children with language impairment, I remain encouraged at our progress. We have documented the reality and extent of their cognitive deficits, and in so doing have validated the inherent connectedness of language and thought. To borrow from Farb (1974), 'language so interpenetrates the experience of being human that neither language nor behavior can be understood without knowledge of both'. The work of the past decade has proven that children with specific language impairment belong to this same human world. To understand their learning patterns and life experiences, we must study both their language and their thought. If our initial attempts to explain language impairment have fallen short, we should be neither surprised nor discouraged, for the scope of our inquiry has become the mind itself.

# References

ALLPORT, A. (1989). Visual attention. In: M. Posner (Ed), *Foundations of Cognitive Science*. Cambridge, Mass: MIT Press.

BATES, E., BENIGNI, L., BRETHERTON, I., CAMAIONI, L. and VOLTERRA, V. (1979). *The Emergence of Symbols: Cognition and Communication in Infancy*. New York: Academic.

BISHOP, D. (1991). The underlying nature of specific language impairment. *Journal of Child Psychology and Psychiatry*, 35, 3–66.

BLOOM, L., MILLER, P. and HOOD, L. (1975). Variation and reduction as aspects of competence in language development. In: A. Pick (Ed.), *Minnesota Symposia on Child Psychology*. Minneapolis: University of Minnesota Press.

BROWN, J., REDMOND, A., BASS, K., LIEBERGOTT, J. and SWOPE, S. (1975). Symbolic play in normal and language impaired children. Paper presented to the American Speech Language Hearing Association.

CAMARATA, S., NEWHOFF, M. and RUGG, B. (1981). Perspective taking in normal and language disordered children. *Proceedings of the Symposium of Research in Child Language Disorders*, 2, 81–88.

CAMARATA, S., NEWHOFF, M. and RUGG, B. (1985). Classification skills and language development in language impaired children. *Australian Journal of Human Communication Disorders*, 13, 107–115.

CECI, S. (1983). Automatic and purposive semantic processing characteristics of normal and language/learning disabled children. *Developmental Psychology*, 19, 427–439.

CHI, M. and GALLAGHER J. (1982). Speed of processing: a developmental source of limitation. *Topics in Learning and Learning Disabilities*, 2, 23–32.

CLAHSEN, H. (1989). The grammatical characterization of developmental aphasia, *Linguistics*, 27, 897–920.

CROMER, R. (1983) Hierarchical planning disability in the drawings and constructions of a special group of severely aphasic children. *Brain and Cognition*, 2, 144-164.

DOEHRING, D. (1960). Visual spatial memory in aphasic children. *Journal of Speech and Hearing Research*, 3, 138–149.

EISENSON, J. (1968) Developmental aphasia: A postulation of a unitary concept of the disorder. *Cortex*, 4, 184-200.

FARB, P. (1974). *Word Play: What happens when People Talk*. New York: Knopf.

INHELDER, B. (1976). Observations on the operational and figurative aspects of thought in dysphasic children. In: D. Morehead and A. Morehead (Eds), *Normal and Deficient Child Language*. Baltimore: University Park Press.

JOHNSTON, J. (1988) Specific language disorders in the child. In: N. Lass, L. McReynolds, J. Northern and D. Yoder (Eds), *Handbook of Speech-Language Pathology and Audiology*. Toronto: B.C.Decker.

JOHNSTON, J. and ELLIS WEISMER, S. (1983). Mental rotation abilities in language disordered children. *Journal of Speech and Hearing Research*, 26, 397–403.

JOHNSTON, J. and RAMSTAD, V. (1983). Cognitive development in pre-adolescent language impaired children. *British Journal of Disorders of Communication*, **18**, 49–55.

JOHNSTON, J. and SMITH, L. (1988). Six ways to skin a cat: Communication strategies used by language impaired preschoolers. Paper presented at the Symposium on Research in Child Language Disorders, University of Wisconsin, Madison.

KAIL, R. and BISANZ, J. (1982). Information processing and cognitive development. In: L. Lipsitt and C. Spiker (Ed.), *Advances in Child Development and Behavior, Vol. 17*. New York: Academic.

KAMHI, A. (1981). Nonlinguistic symbolic and conceptual abilities of language-impaired and normally developing children. *Journal of Speech and Hearing Research*, **24**, 446–453.

KIRCHNER, D. and KLATZKY, R. (1985). Verbal rehearsal and memory in language disordered children. *Journal of Speech and Hearing Research*, **28**, 556–564.

KOSSLYN, S. (1980). *Image and Mind*. Cambridge, Mass: Harvard University Press.

KRACKE, I. (1975). Perception of rhythmic sequences by receptive aphasic and deaf children. *British Journal of Disorders of Communication*, **10**, 43–51.

LEONARD, L., STECKOL, K. and SCHWARTZ, R. (1978). Semantic relations and utterance length in child language. In: F. Peng (Ed.), *Language Acquisition and Developmental Kinesics*. Hiroshima: Bunka Hyoron.

LOVELL, K., HOYLE, H. and SIDDALL, M. (1968). A study of some aspects of the play and language of young children with delayed speech. *Journal of Child Psychology, Psychiatry and Allied Disciplines*, **3**, 41–50.

LOWE, M. and COSTELLO, A. (1976). *The Symbolic Play Test*. Windsor: NFER.

MACKWORTH, N., GRANDSTAFF, N. and PRIBRAM, K. (1973). Orientation to pictorial novelty by speech-disordered children. *Neuropsychologia*, **11**, 443–450.

MOORE, M. (1990). Adverbial and inflectional expressions of past time by normal and language impaired children. Unpublished doctoral dissertation, Indiana University, Bloomington.

MOREHEAD, D. (1972). Early grammatical and semantic relations: Some implications for a general representational deficit in linguistically deviant children. *Papers and Reports in Child Language Development*, **4**, 1–12.

NELSON, L., KAMHI, A. and APEL, K. (1987). Cognitive strengths and weaknesses in language impaired children: one more look. *Journal of Speech and Hearing Disorders*, **52**, 36–43.

OLSON, D. (1975). On the relations between spatial and linguistic processes. In: J. Eliot and N. Salkind (Eds), *Children's Spatial Development*. Springfield: Thomas.

PANAGOS, J. and PRELOCK, P. (1982). Phonological constraints on the sentence productions of language-disordered children. *Journal of Speech and Hearing Research*, **25**, 536–547.

PINKER, S. (1989). Language acquisition. In: M. Posner (Ed.), *Foundations of Cognitive Science*. Cambridge, Mass: MIT Press.

ROTH, R. and CLARK, D. (1987). Symbolic play and social participation abilities of language impaired and normally developing children. *Journal of Speech and Hearing Disorders*, **52**, 17–29.

SIEGEL, L., LEES, A., ALLAN, L. and BOLTON, B. (1981). Nonverbal assessment of Piagetian concepts in preschool children with impaired language development. *Educational Psychology*, **1**, 153–158.

SKARAKIS, E. and PRUTTING, C. (1988). Characteristics of symbolic play in language disordered children. *Human Communication*, **12**, 7–18.

SNYDER, L. (1978). Communicative and cognitive abilities and disabilities in the sensorimotor period. *Merrill-Palmer Quarterly*, **24**, 161–180.

TALLAL, P. (1990). Fine-grained discrimination deficits in language-learning impaired children are specific neither to the auditory modality nor to speech perception. *Journal of Speech and Hearing Research*, **33**, 616–617.

TALLAL, P. (1988). Research implication: A perspective. In: R. Stark, P. Tallal and R. McCauley (Eds), *Language, Speech and Reading Disorders in Children*. Boston:College Hill.

TALLAL, P. and PIERCY, M. (1973). Developmental aphasia: Impaired rate of non-verbal processing as a function of sensory modality. *Neuropsychologia*, **11**, 389–398.

TALLAL, P., STARK, R., KALLMAN, C. and MELLITS, D. (1981). A reexamination of some non-verbal perceptual abilities of language impaired and normal children as a function of age and sensory modality. *Journal of Speech and Hearing Research*, **24**, 351–357.

TERRELL, B. and SCHWARTZ, R. (1988). Object transformations in the play of language impaired children. *Journal of Speech and Hearing Disorders,* **53**, 459–466.

TERRELL, B., SCHWARTZ, R., PRELOCK, P. and MESSICK, C. (1984). Symbolic play in normal and language disordered children. *Journal of Speech and Hearing Research*, **27**, 424–429.

THAL, D. and BATES, E. (1988). Language and gesture in late talkers. *Journal of Speech and Hearing Research*, **31**, 115–123.

UDWIN, O. and YULE, W. (1983). Imaginative play in language disordered children. *British Journal of Disorders of Communication*, **18**, 197–205.

WYKE, M. and ASSO, D. (1979). Perception and memory for spatial relations in children with developmental dysphasia. *Neuropsychologia*, **17**, 231–239.

# Part III

# Language Impairment: Cross-cultural Perspectives

# Chapter 9
# Specific language impairment in three languages: some cross-linguistic evidence

LAURENCE B. LEONARD

Many English-speaking children with specific language impairment have mild to moderate deficits in a range of language areas but a more serious problem with morphology. This is typically revealed when English-speaking specifically language-impaired (ESLI) children are compared with a group of younger normally developing children who are matched according to a general measure of language development such as mean length of utterance (MLU). Studies of this type usually report that despite the similar length of sentences in the two groups of children, the ESLI children show less use of inflections (e.g. -s̲,-e̲d̲) and function words (e.g. i̲s̲, t̲h̲e̲).

The purpose of this paper is to discuss several possible reasons for the extraordinary difficulty that morphology seems to present to ESLI children. A cross-linguistic approach is taken, because the natural confounds that exist in English would greatly limit the hypotheses that could be considered if this were the sole source of information. I shall rely on evidence from Italian, as well as some preliminary data from Hebrew. First, I shall review three alternative hypotheses that might account for ESLI children's special problems with morphology. In so doing, I will at the same time note how the inclusion of Italian-speaking (I) SLI children can assist in the evaluation of each hypothesis. A summary of the available evidence from ESLI and ISLI children will then be presented. The alternative hypotheses will then receive a final evaluation using preliminary data obtained from SLI children acquiring Hebrew.

**Three Hypotheses**

*Sparse Morphology Hypothesis*

Although inflections occur in English, nouns, verbs, and adjectives frequently appear as bare stems (e.g. *cars* but also *car, runs* but also *run)*. It seems possible that the paucity of inflections in English might contribute to ESLI children's lack of attention to grammatical morphemes in favor of more dependable cues, such as word order. That is, if ESLI children have limited resources, it may be more adaptive to focus on those aspects of the grammar that are more reliable. We shall refer to this hypothesis as the ' sparse morphology' hypothesis.

Unlike English, Italian is a morphologically rich and uniform language, and nouns, verbs, and adjectives can never appear as bare stems. For example, one can say *scrivo* ' I write,' *scrivi* ' you write,' and *scrive* ' he or she writes,' but never *\*scriv*. Consequently, when an Italian child hears a noun, verb, or adjective, the word is always accompanied by an inflection that modulates its meaning. If a child acquiring this language were faced with limited resources, as presumably is the case for ISLI children, inflections would be the place to focus attention.

Evaluation of the sparse morphology hypothesis requires a two-step process. First, ISLI children should show greater use of grammatical inflections than ESLI children. However, the advantage of an inflectionally rich morphology over an inflectionally sparse morphology probably holds for normally developing children as well. Therefore, to account for ESLI chldren's especially weak morphology, we must also find that the differences between ESLI children and their MLU-matched English-speaking controls are greater than the differences between ISLI children and MLU-matched Italian controls.

*Surface Hypothesis*

Another possible reason for ESLI children's poor morphology is that many of the grammatical morphemes of English might present perceptual and articulatory obstacles that are too difficult for these children to overcome. The grammatical morphemes are difficult perceptually because, as non-syllabic consonant segments and unstressed syllables, they are shorter in duration than adjacent morphemes. From the standpoint of production, they are vulnerable to final consonant deletion and weak syllable deletion.

However, an adequate explanation cannot be based on perceptual and articulatory factors alone, for ESLI children show greater use of the same phonetic forms when these forms appear in non-morphophonemic contexts. For example, higher percentages of use of [t] are seen in *raft* than in *laughed*. A more reasonable proposal is that the perceptual and articulatory characteristics of English grammatical morphemes make ESLI children's task of morphological paradigm building especially difficult. For example, although the perception of [t] in *raft* may be difficult for ESLI children, the acquisition of [t] in *laughed* will be even more problematic because, in the case of the latter, the children must not only perceive [t], they must also relate *laughed* to *laugh*, and place *laughed* in the appropriate cell of a morphological paradigm (see Pinker, 1984). It is possible that these operations severely tax the resources of SLI children when coupled with the already greater perceptual demands placed upon them by the surface properties of these morphemes. As a result, the demanding morphemes would be slow in entering and becoming established in the paradigm of each word, yielding the findings of less frequent use of grammatical morphemes by ESLI children than by MLU-matched controls. Hereafter, we shall refer to this hypothesis as the 'surface' hypothesis.

Italian differs from English in that many grammatical morphemes take the form of word-final vowels or word-final multisyllabic morphemes ending in vowels. Most of these morphemes do not receive primary stress, but, because Italian has relatively flexible word order, all of these word-final syllabic morphemes can appear in clause-final position, and hence benefit from clause-final vowel lengthening. According to the surface hypothesis, then, ISLI children should use these morphemes to the same degree as their MLU-matched compatriots. An additional test of this hypothesis is permitted because there are also several morphemes in Italian that resemble those seen in English, taking the form of unstressed syllables whose vowels are not in a position to receive lengthening. These particular morphemes should be produced with lower percentages by the ISLI children than by their MLU-matched controls.

### Missing Feature Hypothesis

The third and final hypothesis to be considered stems from the recent work of Gopnik (1990a, 1990b). She has proposed that some SLI children's extraordinary difficulties with grammatical morphology might be due to the absence of syntactico-semantic features in their underlying grammars. Because these features are absent, both morphophonemic rules as well as rules that match features in the syntax will be missing. Consequently, in a deficit of this type there would be no feature marking for number, person, tense, and aspect. This is not to say that the child will never produce a form that resembles plural -s or past -ed. However, in such instances the form would either be an unanalysed portion of a memorised lexical item, or would be in free variation with the bare stem and not reflect an underlying feature. This proposal shall be referred to as the ' missing feature' hypothesis.

This hypothesis can be tested quite easily in Italian. There are several grammatical morphemes in the language whose appropriate use clearly requires the presence of features in the underlying grammar, yet they pose no special difficulty in terms of their perceptual and articulatory characteristics. These include verb inflections that must agree with the subject in person and number, and adjective endings that must agree with the noun in number and gender. According to the missing feature hypothesis, all morphemes of this type should be more difficult for ISLI children than for MLU-matched controls.

## Evaluating the Hypotheses

### Some Data from English

Before turning to data from Italian and Hebrew, we consider first some data from English. We review here a recent study by Leonard et al. (1990). Two of the subject groups in that study were 10 ESLI children ranging in age from 3;8 to 5;7 and in MLU in words from 2.7 to 4.2, and 10 normally developing children matched with the ESLI children according to MLU (hereafter, END-MLU children). This second group ranged in age from 2;11 to 3;4 and in MLU from 2.9 to 4.2 words. Spontaneous speech samples were obtained from each child, but to ensure a sufficient number of obligatory contexts for the grammatical morphemes of interest, preselected pictures were also presented. A summary of the children's use of the grammatical morphemes appears in Table 9.1.

**Table 9.1** Summary of the English-speaking children's production of grammatical morphemes in obligatory contexts

|                 | ESLI | END-MLU |
|-----------------|------|---------|
| Articles        | 52   | 62      |
| Plurals         | 69   | 96      |
| Third singular  | 34   | 59      |
| Regular past    | 32   | 65      |
| Irregular past  | 65   | 77      |
| Copula          | 41   | 71      |

All values are mean percentages.

Full interpretation of these data must await presentation of the findings from Italian, but it can be noted at this point that the percentages shown in Table 9.1 are equally compatible with the surface and the missing feature hypotheses. According to the former, all of the grammatical morphemes except the irregular past should be problematic because they involve final consonants or unstressed syllables. Because the irregular past involves, at a minimum, a vowel change in a stressed syllable, it should not create special problems for the ESLI children. In the case of the missing feature hypothesis, all of the grammatical morphemes except the irregular past require underlying features. The irregular past, in contrast, can be learned as a lexical item.

The ESLI and END-MLU children did not differ in their use of the irregular past; the numerical difference shown in Table 9.1 did not achieve statistical significance. But neither did the difference seen for articles, a finding that runs counter to the predictions of both of these hypotheses. For the remaining grammatical morphemes, the percentages of use seen for the END-MLU children were in fact higher than those for the ESLI children, and thus supported each of the two hypotheses.

### Data from Italian

Two other subject groups in the Leonard et al. (1990) study were Italian-speaking children: 15 ISLI children ranging in age from 4;0 to 6;0 and in MLU in words from 1.9 to 4.3, and 15 normally developing children matched with the ISLI children according to MLU (the IND-MLU children). This latter group ranged in age from 2;6 to 3;6 and in MLU in words from 2.1 to 4.3. The data collection procedures matched those used with the English-speaking children. The grammatical morphemes of interest are provided in Table 9.2, and a summary of the children's use of these morphemes can be seen in Table 9.3.

From the standpoint of the surface hypothesis, articles and clitics are expected to be difficult for ISLI children because they are unstressed syllables that do not receive vowel lengthening (clitics were assessed only in clause-medial position). The remaining grammatical morphemes should be relatively easy for the ISLI children, as they involve word-

**Table 9.2** Some Italian grammatical morphemes examined by Leonard et al., 1990

| Grammatical morpheme | Example |
| --- | --- |
| Article | la chiave, il pane |
| Plural | gatti, stelle |
| Third singular | legge, compra |
| Noun-adjective agreement | chiave piccola, cane piccolo |
| Clitics | Gina lo vede 'Gina sees him' |

**Table 9.3** Summary of the Italian-speaking children's production of grammatical morphemes

|                | ISLI | IND-MLU |
|----------------|------|---------|
| Articles       | 41   | 83      |
| Plurals        | 87   | 89      |
| Third singular | 93   | 93      |
| Noun-adjective | 97   | 99      |
| Clitics        | 26   | 66      |

All values are mean percentages.

final vowels that can be lengthened. According to the missing feature hypothesis, the ISLI children should have greater difficulty than the IND-MLU children with all of these grammatical morphemes, because each requires a feature presumed missing from the children's grammars. Finally, the sparse morphology hypothesis predicts that those grammatical inflections occurring in both Italian and English will be produced with higher percentages by the Italian children and that the differences between SLI and ND-MLU children will be larger in English.

Two of the grammatical morphemes, the noun plural and the third person singular verb inflection, were examined in both English and Italian and can be used to evaluate the sparse morphology hypothesis. The first test in this two-step evaluation produced results that were in keeping with the hypothesis: A comparison of the English and Italian data in Tables 9.1 and 9.3 shows that percentages for the plural and the third person singular were higher for the ISLI children. The second step, too, yielded results that were favourable for the hypothesis. Specifically, the differences between the ISLI and IND-MLU children in the use of these two morphemes were smaller than the differences between the ESLI and END-MLU children. This can be seen clearly from Tables 9.1 and 9.3.

The findings for Italian were also supportive of the surface hypothesis. According to this hypothesis, the ISLI children should show lower percentages than the IND-MLU children only on the article and clitics. Precisely this pattern was observed.

The missing feature hypothesis did not fare as well. In particular, for three of the grammatical morphemes that seemingly required features – noun plurals, third person singular verb inflections, and noun-adjective agreement – the ISLI children's use did not differ from that of the IND-MLU children. Furthermore, the fact that the percentages for these particular morphemes were so high makes it unlikely that they were the result of the memorization of individual lexical items.

*Preliminary Data from Hebrew*

Like Italian, Hebrew has a rich morphology in which nouns, adjectives, and verbs are always inflected. However, unlike Italian, in which the stem is almost always readily identifiable, the base unit in Hebrew is a tri-consonantal root. In some cases, grammatical distinctions are made by the addition of a suffix, in others they are made by word-internal vowel changes, and in the bulk of cases, they are made by changes in both a suffix and a vowel. For example, the verb 'finish' has the root *g-m-r*. 'He finishes' has the form *gomer*, 'she finishes' has the form *gomeret*, 'he finished' has the form *gamar*, and 'they finished' has the form *gamru*. (Hebrew examples are written in phonemic notation rather than Hebrew script for clarity of presentation.)

Because nouns, verbs, and adjectives are always inflected, the sparse morphology hypothesis would predict that Hebrew-speaking (H)SLI children would show greater use of bound morphemes than their English-speaking counterparts, and the difference between HSLI children and HND-MLU children would be smaller than the difference between ESLI and END-MLU children. According to the surface hypothesis, these same bound morphemes would not be any more difficult for HSLI children than for their MLU controls, because these morphemes are syllabic and receive either primary stress or vowel lengthening in clause-final position. On the other hand, certain free-standing morphemes are unstressed syllables that never benefit from vowel lengthening. For these morphemes, HSLI children should show percentages of use below those of HND-MLU children. The predictions of the missing feature hypothesis are quite different. Because all of these morphemes can be presumed to require features such as number, gender, and definiteness in the underlying grammar, they should be especially difficult for HSLI children.

Only preliminary evidence from Hebrew is available at this point. These data come from a study by Rom and Leonard (1990). The subjects were seven HSLI children ranging in age from 4;4 to 5;3 and in MLU in words from 1.8 to 3.4, and seven normally developing children who served as MLU controls (HND-MLU children). This second group of children ranged in age from 2;4 to 3;3 and in MLU from 1.8 to 3.3 words. Spontaneous speech samples served as the source of data. Because these samples were relatively short, it was necessary to collapse some of the specific grammatical morphemes into a single category (e.g. past inflections). The grammatical morphemes of interest appear in Table 9.4, and the results can be found in Table 9.5.

As can be seen from Table 9.5, the HSLI children's percentages of use were equivalent to those of the HND-MLU children for all of the

**Table 9.4** Some Hebrew grammatical morphemes examined by Rom and Leonard (1990)

| Grammatical morpheme | Example |
|---|---|
| Plural | iton<u>im</u>, dir<u>ot</u> |
| Noun–adjective agreement | bait gadol, mexonit gdola |
| Present inflections | holex, holxot |
| Past inflections | halax, halxa, halxu |
| Accusative case marker | hu ohev et Rina: 'he loves Rina' |

The 'x' in Hebrew has the sound of 'ch' in loch.

grammatical inflections, but not for the unstressed free-standing marker *et*. These findings are entirely consistent with the surface hypothesis, but inconsistent with the missing feature hypothesis. The sparse morphology hypothesis also receives support from these findings. First, it can be seen from a comparison of Table 9.5 and Table 9.1 that the HSLI children showed higher percentages than the ESLI children for the inflections of plural, present (in English, third singular), and past. Second, the differences between the ESLI and END-MLU children were much larger than the (nonexistent) differences between the HSLI and HND-MLU children.

**Table 9.5** Summary of the Hebrew-speaking children's production of grammatical morphemes

|  | HSLI | HND-MLU |
|---|---|---|
| Plurals | 100 | 100 |
| Noun-adjective | 74 | 75 |
| Present inflections | 94 | 97 |
| Past inflections | 93 | 89 |
| Accusative case marker | 64 | 94 |

All values are mean percentages.

### Summary

Although it is highly possible that there are children whose underlying grammars lack features, this characterisation does not seem appropriate for the children described here. For these children, two other accounts seem more plausible. The first of these holds that SLI children acquiring English do not direct their limited resources toward the relatively sparse morphological information that is available in the ambient language. The second states that the challenging perceptual and/or articulatory characteristics of English grammatical morphemes exceed the limited resources of SLI children when combined with the task of morphological paradigm building. It is not clear which, if either, of these accounts will prove correct. However, it does appear that the answer will come more quickly if we take advantage of the natural separation of confounding factors that is afforded by including languages other than English in our research.

## References

GOPNIK, M. (1990a). Feature-blind grammar and dysphasia. *Nature, 344*, 715.

GOPNIK, M. (1990b). Feature blindness: A case study. *Language Acquisition, 1*, 139–164.

LEONARD, L., BORTOLINI, U., CASELLI, M. C. and MCGREGOR, K. (1990). Two accounts of morphological deficits in children with specific language impairment. *Language Aquisition* (in press).

PINKER, S. (1984). *Language Learnability and Language Development*. Cambridge, MA: Harvard University Press.

ROM, A. and LEONARD, L. (1990). Interpreting deficits in grammatical morphology in specifically language-impaired children: Preliminary evidence from Hebrew. *Clinical Linguistics and Pnonetics, 4*, 93–105.

# Chapter 10
# Child language impairment in the Hong Kong context

ANN ZUBRICK

## Background

In September 1988 the Department of Speech and Hearing Sciences was established in the University of Hong Kong. The mission of the department includes the education of speech and language therapists (especially to overcome the shortage in Hong Kong) and the study of speech and hearing disorders in Chinese. The department is the first to undertake such studies systematically as its primary focus of research, and the degree programmes offered are the only ones which provide studies in clinical linguistics in Chinese. Given that Chinese is the language of one-quarter of the world's population, we know remarkably little about either its acquisition or how persons are affected in their processing or production when they have speech and language disorders. As a tonal and logographic language Chinese affords opportunities to test out models and theories in some interesting and informative ways. Cantonese, the dialect of Chinese used by the majority of people in Hong Kong and adjacent Guandong province, is spoken by at least 56 million people in Hong Kong and China, and many more if expatriate Chinese are included. Currently there is only fragmentary published data on a few select aspects of Cantonese linguistics appearing in sources such as the *Journal of Chinese Linguistics*. A small number of articles both on language acquisition and aphasia (mostly in Mandarin speakers) have appeared in international journals with a wider readership. Much basic descriptive research remains to be done.

The task of the Department has been to develop a 4-year undergraduate curriculum which allows graduates to practise speech therapy in both English and Cantonese Chinese. With the advent of Hong Kong's return to Chinese rule in 1997, the curriculum may be extended to include Mandarin Chinese also. The academic courses are taught in English while the practice contexts are mostly Cantonese. Not uncommonly, clients or members of their family speak other dialects of Chinese such as Mandarin, Fukinese, Shanghainese etc.

Speech therapy has a relatively short history in Hong Kong. Most of the 30 or so Cantonese-speaking practitioners qualified less than 5 years ago in a variety of English-speaking programmes. The graduates therefore returned to Hong Kong without a background in Chinese linguistics and with little formal study which prepared them for the contrasts in practice found in Hong Kong. Practising clinicians frequently comment on the difficulty of applying concepts learnt in other contexts to speech and language disorders in Cantonese. Native-speaker proficiency is not a substitute for specific linguistic studies, especially when the languages are as different as English and Chinese. So, in these beginning years of the Department's work the task is to equip the students to study normal and abnormal speech and language in Cantonese Chinese, as a basis for applying this knowledge within their local environment, as well as to begin the task of systematically describing the features of speech and language disability in Chinese. A group of 11 Chinese and Western teachers have begun this work, much of which will be developed by the graduates of the programme. Because of the short time frame since the work began, I can report only on preliminary findings and observations and suggest some ways in which it may be informative to look at speech and language disorders in Chinese cross linguistic contexts. Some brief descriptions of Cantonese and the language-learning environment of Hong Kong as background.

**Features of Cantonese**

Cantonese is a tonal language. This means that tone operates lexically to change meanings. Lexical tone is defined as the use of fundamental frequency to distinguish minimal word pairs that are not differentiated by segmental information (Baudion-Chial, 1986). Cantonese has six primary tones (Fok, 1974) and three entering tones. A segmental phonology test on Cantonese must therefore include information on consonants, vowels and tones. Some segmental units (such as those in the examples given below) show all the possible tone contrasts.

|  | high falling | high rising | high level | low falling | low rising | low level |
|---|---|---|---|---|---|---|
| /ji/ | 1 | 2 | 3 | 4 | 5 | 6 |
|  | cure | chair | opinion | son | ear | two |
| /fu/ | husband | tiger | trousers | holding | woman | father |

Studies of tone acquisition show that the tones of both Mandarin and Cantonese are acquired very early, earlier than the segmentals (Li and Thompson, 1977), and that tones are highly salient to the child. When infants aged 12–15 months were given tasks where there was a mismatch between the tonal and segmental information, these young Cantonese-speaking children attended to the tonal rather than the segmental information (So, 1989).

However, children do make tonal errors in production which they recognise and repair in their conversational speech. How early this metalinguistic behaviour occurs is not yet known. Nor do we know if it occurs with all tones or only a subset of them. Fok (1974) found in her tone-perception studies that adults confused tones with similar 'frequency patterns.Thus the rising tones were confused with each other, as were the falling tones with level tones, since level tones do in fact fall slightly. These sorts of problems do not usually arise in conversational speech since contexts give clues to meanings where meanings may be ambiguous. Furthermore, words are usually not produced in isolation as was the case in Fok's study. Tone contrasts are particularly difficult to hear when words are said in isolation; a finding which has particular implications both for the development of tests (such as naming pictures to test phonology or lexical knowledge) and the use of certain types of metalinguistic activities in speech therapy .

**The Importance of Tone in Comprehension**

What role does tone play in comprehension? In conversation the importance of tone is reduced because of the contribution of context. However, Fok's research (Fok, 1984,1987) has indicated that tonal information is particularly important in noisy situations. In sentences with tonal variation, high levels of intelligibility are reached even when signal-to-noise ratios are increased. By contrast, in monotoned sentences, the degree of intelligibility with similar signal-to-noise ratios is reduced from 45% to only 17%. Furthermore in ordinary conversational speech, co-articulatory effects affect the vowels and consonants (the segmental features) but tone remains intrinsic, subject to predictable changes.

Hearing-impaired Chinese-speaking children appear to be significantly advantaged in acquiring a tonal language. The lexical information available to them through tones occurs in the frequency range of 500 Hz and below. Consequently even profoundly hearing-impaired children have access to considerable linguistic (lexical) information (Clezy, 1990). Clezy has observed that Chinese-speaking hearing-impaired children develop more normal voice patterns including stress, pitch, duration and rhythm in their speech. As yet there are no longitudinal studies of how these features emerge in the speech of hearing-impaired children. However, if this observation is supported empirically in subsequent studies it may be an important finding, especially for children growing up in a bilingual environment. The child may have an advantage in an aural–oral approach if the first spoken language is tonal.

Processing of lexical tones appears to be left hemisphere based and tonal information appears to be coded together with lexical information. Consequently, tonal comprehension might well be affected with left hemisphere lesions. This has indeed been found true for adult aphasics, regardless of the type of aphasia (Yiu, 1989). Paraphasic tone errors occurred on word repetition tasks in Chinese aphasic subjects with left hemisphere lesions (Packard 1984,1986). Moreover, these tone errors occurred with about the same frequency as segmental errors. It will be important to keep these findings in mind as opportunities arise to study children with acquired speech and language disorders. From such children it should be possible to investigate how tonal information is related to lexical and phonological processing and production during development, as well as to study the sequence of recovery.

### The Structure of Chinese

A syllable in Chinese consists of both segmental and suprasegmental features. The segmental features of Cantonese include 17 consonants and two consonant clusters, together with vowels, diphthongs and triphthongs. The suprasegmental features include the distinctive tones that are part of the phonological components of the syllables. A segmental phonological assessment in Chinese therefore has to include consonants, vowels and tones. Phonemes and tonemes are linguistically contrastive.

Cantonese has a simpler syllable structure than English. Most syllables are either C, CV or CVC structure. Whilst English is a stress timed language in which different syllables within a word have different stress, Cantonese is syllable timed with syllables occurring at regular intervals.

At present there is very little data on the acquisition of Cantonese phonology. However, So (1992) has produced a pilot phonological assessment and normative data are being collected. So far tasks of stimulability of isolated phonemes are proving to be difficult for Cantonese speakers. Syllables appear to be coded as a single unit. Initial sound cues do not act as triggers to word production. The learning of a logographic writing system does not help to make transparent the relationships of sounds to words as is the case in alphabetic scripts. Phonological metalinguistic ability is likely to be quite different among

Chinese children. Currently some studies are under way to further examine metalinguistic knowledge about tones, phonemes and syllables in child and adult speakers.

Cantonese is fundamentally a subject–verb–object (SVO) language that lacks an inflectional morphology. One might be tempted to assume that such a language would be easier to acquire since acquisition would largely rest on semantics. As Erbaugh (1992) points out, if this were true, then Chinese children should not only learn their language very rapidly, but they should show few errors. The acquisition data do not bear this out and the data show error patterns and rules analogous in principle to those made by European children.

Morphological markers in Chinese nouns are used for classification, qualification and quantification; those with verbs mark negation, aspect and interrogatives. There are complex psycholinguistic rules governing the use of such markers. These rules must be well understood before one can decide whether usage of these particles is normal or reflects linguistic breakdown or misuse of some kind. This is especially true in Cantonese which is much less formal than other forms of Chinese and where the use of markers is not necessarily obligatory. Non-obligatory and flexible use of forms create particular difficulties for language analysis and in the design of tasks to tap usage. It will take some considerable work, especially in sociolinguistics, to define acceptable uses of forms by adult and child speakers against which relevant comparisons of disordered usage can be made. It may also be the case that young Cantonese-speaking children who have a reasonable grasp of the semantic system are not readily identified as language disordered at an early age. Developmental errors in the use of aspect markers or classifiers (both complex systems to acquire) may be tolerated if the overall meaning is generally clear. This hypothesis has yet to be tested.

## Pragmatic Rules

The pragmatic rules governing usage of Cantonese are different from those of English. Chinese children are taught to be humble. When given praise, they are often embarrassed and rejecting of compliments. Where in Western cultures one is taught to accept compliments graciously, in Chinese one dismisses one's own achievements or those of close family members. Children do not ask many questions, at least in instructional contexts. Within Chinese culture interruption through the asking of questions during classes or during exchnages with people perceived to be of high status is considered rude. By Western standards, children may appear more passive and non-participative. They will wait for the adult to initiate and to define the rules for that context. Children who break these rules, even when they are only infants, may be described by their parents as 'naughty'. On the whole, new situations are treated more formally. Three year olds are quite willing to sit at a table and attend to routine and repetitive tasks for lengthy stretches of 20 minutes or more. They are well socialised from an early age to contexts of formal instruction.

Therapy which is geared around following the child's lead and which asks caregivers to take a child-directed focus operates counter to more traditional teaching styles. Erbaugh (1992) describes the 'Quiz Style' of conversation as the normal one adopted by older children and adults talking with young children. The quiz style is analogous to display questioning techniques where an adult asks the child a question to which there is an expected answer and then persists in asking the same question until the child produces exactly the answer required. The quiz style of talk is adopted at about the time that the child begins to use single words and persists through teachers' talk in the school years. Answers which do not conform with what is expected are labelled as disorderly behaviour. Clearly it is important to understand the impact of this style when considering the management of children who have a limited linguistic repertoire and who may not be able to produce required responses. Yet intervention approaches which run counter to the natural interactive patterns of caregivers may not be used outside the clinical context. The quiz style of interaction best prepares the children for the realities of the Chinese school system which stresses conformity, uniform responses and high degrees of memorisation. Success at school is highly valued. The quiz style of interaction provides children with many opportunities to learn names, appropriate comments and greetings and politeness forms. It takes place in relaxed settings in which there are many social rewards for responding successfully.

Different social rules apply to the asking of quesions and the giving of comments. Because of the status accorded to age, it is not considered rude to ask people how old they are. Comments are freely given about people's size or weight, even in very public forums.

Clearly it is important to understand the different rules which apply to the structure and use of Cantonese as a framework against which to make judgements about disordered language performance. Such information is not only important for work in a first language context, but also to those professionals who see Chinese children and their families in North America, Australasia or Europe.

## The Language-learning Environment of Hong Kong Children

Hong Kong currently has a population of 5.8 million inhabitants, 98% of whom are Chinese. The remaining 2% are expatriates comprising

Filipino migrant workers, British, European, North American and Australasian business and professional people attracted by opportunities in their respective fields. Despite more than 100 years of British colonial rule, Hong Kong remains essentially a Cantonese-speaking community in which some English is spoken for official and business purposes. English has currency as an international language but its value is reduced because it is a colonial language. In many families, more than one Chinese 'dialect' is spoken. With the advent of Chinese rule in 1997 Putonghua (literally 'the peoples's language' and a form of Chinese derived from Mandarin) is gaining increasing importance.

The sociolinguistic context in which young Hong Kong children learn to speak is complex. The parental/home language is largely Cantonese but may include other forms of Chinese depending upon the family origin and composition. Grandparents may well speak only the form of Chinese they learned as children in their home provinces, rather than Cantonese. If the family has a live-in maid, and many do, she is likely to be Filipina or Thai. She will speak to the children in her care in English or her own native language. The maid, the grandmother and the mother may all share caregiving and, consequently, the child may be exposed to several languages simultaneously.

Once young children enter kindergarten at age 3 years, they are introduced to both basic Chinese characters and the English alphabet through quite formal processes of instruction. At primary school the medium of instruction is overwhelmingly Cantonese but English is taught as a subject in many primary schools. However, the dearth of qualified language teachers results in Cantonese being used extensively even in 'English' classes and mixed-code teaching predominates into high school. The text and reference books as well as key terms in the subject areas may be in English, but the oral language of the classroom is essentially Cantonese. Once outside the business and tourist areas of Hong Kong, little English is used.

Young Cantonese speakers learning to read and write Chinese face many challenges. Modern Standard Chinese (based on Mandarin) is the language used for writing and has its traditions in the language of scholars. Its history dates back to ancient texts. Cantonese historically is a spoken language of traders and peasants. It is a casual, street dialect of exchanges and is highly colloquial, changes rapidly and uses common lexical items in humorous ways. Puns are especially liked. By comparison, it has simplified some of its structures in ways appropriate for informal exchanges.

Cantonese children learning to read and write have to learn the formal language of written texts, based on Mandarin, which differs significantly from their spoken language. This form of Chinese (Modern

Standard Chinese) is rarely used orally, except for formal exchanges such as radio reports (Bauer, 1988) and differs from colloquial Cantonese lexically, grammatically and in its formalisms. Unlike spoken Cantonese, it is liable to much less change. In moving to reading and writing, children have to adopt a much more formal code in which word order, grammatical markers and even changes in the lexicon have to be learned and strictly observed. For example, the young child will first hear and learn the phonetic sequence /tsʰɛ / for the word umbrella. When the child encounters the same concept in print the Modern Standard Chinese character is pronounced as /ji saŋ/. Later, in more informal contexts employing written Cantonese (such as might be found in a small restaurant or shop) the child will see a quite unfamiliar character corresponding to phonetic form /tsʰɛ /.

Unfortunately even native speakers of Cantonese do not understand these differences between the spoken and written forms and the contexts of use very well. Indeed many teachers are totally unable to explain what the differences are. This lack of knowledge must have an inpact on the quality and type of classroom instruction given to young readers and writers. The didactic teaching methods which employ extensive repetition and drilling proably result in children learning the differences, but not in them understanding how the forms relate. For children with significant language disorders, one might anticipate considerable difficulties in moving from one system to another. On the other hand the invariant methods of repetitive instruction may have some advantages for these children.

Learning to read and write is a mammoth task. Chinese represents every word by an ideograph or character, sometimes by two or more and one needs to recognise at least 2000 of them to be able to read a simple book or newspaper article and many more to cope with less common words. Characters contain two parts; one is a phonetic element which gives a clue as to the pronunciation, and the other is a radical, which gives the semantic element. A knowledge of the phonetic components makes it possible to pronounce a great many new words. Similarly some 80% of words contain one of 214 radicals. Words that are related in meaning usually contain the same radical. However a great deal of time is required to recognise and write the radicals. Consequently Chinese children must go through repeated practice and lengthy periods of homework. Learning to read and write taxes visual memory in different ways from learning an alphabetic system of only 26 letters. Children have to give close attention to fine detail and the visual–spatial relationships among the components. The little work that has so far been done on reading disability among Chinese children shows that children have more difficulty with the radical components than with the phonetic ones (Hoosain, 1986). As detailed work is undertaken on types of child language disorders, it will be useful to see how children with different types of phonological and semantic disorders proceed to learn the two components and the types of errors that they make in doing so.

### Implications for Studying Disorders in Chinese Children

The study of disorders in cross-linguistic and cross-cultural settings allows assumptions to be tested in systematic ways. I have already suggested some phemomena which might be examined in Cantonese-speaking children and I expect that some of the data necessary for defining further questions will become available over the next few years. Much will rely on normative studies. For example, we need to know more about the nature of normally occurring tone confusions in young children to learn how tone is related to other aspects of the phonological system. When do normal children show errors on tone and how long do these errors persist?. It is likely that there will be errors where tone interacts with the semantic system in less obvious ways such as when tone changes lexemes from one grammatical category to another. Tone changing nouns to verb (seed to plant) or directionality (buy to sell) would be examples here. Tonal changes also mark adjectival contrasts (big and small) and status (friend to just chap). Sometimes these status differences can be acheived grammatically as well as through tone. Which alternative do young children use as part of their system and when do they understand that there is a choice? Do language-disordered children find it easier or harder to manipulate tonal than other semantic or syntactic contrasts? Findings from such studies would usefully inform understandings of language and language disability.

English-speaking children show features of specific language disability in the acquisition of grammatical morphemes. In Chinese children we should expect to see patterns of disability in the use of aspect markers for verbs and classifiers for nouns but not in particles which have a highly regular use such as question particles or negatives. Classifiers are a potentially rich source of information about the nature of semantic categories, over-generalisation and over-marking since some things have inherent classifiers and do not require specification. Verbs in Chinese have no tense, no person or number and no active/passive differences.The aspectual contrasts are complex. Erbaugh (1992) notes that young Mandarin speakers suffixed verb aspect to adverbs (evidence of the difficulty they may have in distinguishing between the two classes) and only slowly worked out ways to express temporal contrasts through aspectual distinctions. However, young children did show a sensitivity to inherent semantic verb features in what they chose to mark. In Cantonese the colloquial uses of language result in aspectual distinctions being less obligatory in their marking than in Mandarin. Consequently more data will be needed relating forms to contexts of use before the developmental data can be easily interpreted. It may be some time before it is possible to accurately describe disorders in aspectual use in Cantonese.

## Summary

The context for teaching and developing speech and hearing sciences in Hong Kong is a complex one. It is not clear to what extent models and frameworks derived from data on normal and disordered English speakers will transfer into a Chinese context. The potential is enormous. There are many ways to collect data on a given area. One hopes that the results of these various research endeavours will converge, but where they do not they should provide rich insights into our misperceptions and fragmentary understandings. Making sense of cross-linguistic and cross-cultural research is a risky undertaking but the scientific journey is worth it.

## Ackowledgements

I could not have written this paper without the insights I have gained in discussion with staff and students in the Department of Speech and Hearing Sciences. I thank them for their endless patience and help in coming to understand, in my simple way, the richness of a language whose roots stretch back 3500 years.

## References

BAUDION-CHIAL, S. (1986). Hemispheric lateralisation of Modern Standard Chinese tone processes. *Journal of Neurolinguistics*, 2, 189–199.

BAUER, R. (1988). Written Cantonese of Hong Kong. *Cahiers de Linguistique Asie Orientale*, 17, 2445–293

CLEZY, G. (1990). Management of hearing impairment in young children. Paper presented to the 6th Asian Regional Conference of Rehabilitation International, Beijing, China, November.

ERBAUGH, M. (1992).The acquisition of Mandarin. In: D.I.Slobin (Ed.), *The Cross-linguistic Study of Language Acquisition*. Volume 3. Hillsdale, New Jersey:Lawrence Erlbaum (in press).

FOK, A.Y.Y. (1974). *A Perceptual Study of Tone in Cantonese*. Hong Kong: Hong Kong University Press.

FOK, A.Y.Y. (1984). The teaching of tones to children with profound hearing impairment. *British Journal of Disorders of Communication*, 19, 225–236.

FOK, A.Y.Y. (1987). A study of the part tones play in determining the comprehension threshold of Cantonese. Paper presented to the First International Conference on Cantonese and Yue dialects. Chinese University of Hong Kong, November.

HOOSAIN, R. (1986). Chinese cognition. In: M. Bond (Ed.), *The Psychology of the Chinese People*. Hong Kong: Oxford University Press.

LI, C.N. and THOMPSON, S.A. (1977). The acquisition of tone in Mandarin-speaking children. *Journal of Child Language*, 4, 185–199.

PACKARD, J.L. (1984). *A linguistic investigation of tone lateralisation in aphasic Chinese speakers*. Unpublished PhD dissertation, Cornell University.

PACKARD, J.L.(1986). Tone production deficits in non-fluent aphasic Chinese speech. *Brain and Language*, 29, 212–223.

SO, L.K.H.C. (1989). Tone acquisition in Cantonese-speaking children. Seminar presented at the University of Hong Kong, March.

SO, L.K.H.C. (1992). Cantonese phonological assessment. (Pilot version available through the Department of Speech and Hearing Sciences, University of Hong Kong).

YIU, E. (1989). *Tone perception in Cantonese aphasics*. Unpublished MPhil thesis, University of Hong Kong.

# Chapter 11
# Language impairment in Swedish children: a multidisciplinary approach

ULRIKA NETTELBLADT

## Introduction

The major part of the research in specific language impairment in children has until now focused on American or British English. It is possible that some basic assumptions on what constitutes the linguistic characteristics of language impairment in children may be invalid when confronted with data from other languages. It is thus welcome that there has been an increased interest in cross-linguistic comparisons of children with language impairment in recent years (Leonard et al., 1987, and Leonard, this volume). Important research questions are whether children with different mother tongues share some universal linguistic tendencies, or if they exhibit different language profiles as a function of specific linguistic characteristics of the individual languages involved. The present research can be placed within this emerging research tradition, since it is based on Swedish children with language impairment.

To assist the reader unacquainted with Swedish, a brief survey will be given of some important linguistic characteristics to be mastered by learners of this language. The focus will be on grammatical, phonological and prosodic phenomena. Swedish is a Germanic language, belonging to the Scandinavian language family. Compared with English, Swedish grammar is more inflected but is less inflected than German. Problems with word order is one of the more common errors in children with grammatical disability (Hansson, 1991; Hansson and Nettelbladt, 1991) and, interestingly enough, word order also presents a long-lasting problem for learners of Swedish as a second language (Håkansson, 1988). In topicalised sentences, i.e. with a sentence element other than the subject placed sentence-initially, there is obligatory inverted word order, which means that the finite verb always has to come as the second element.

Related to word order is the position of negation which is different in main and subordinate clauses. As shown by Hyltenstam (1977) second language learners of Swedish pass through distinct developmental stages of negation. In the early stages negation is always placed preverbally and it is not until the latest stage that the learner is able to place the negation correctly in auxiliary contexts in subordinate clauses. Preliminary findings suggest that the developmental order of placement of negation is the same for language-impaired children as for second language learners, (Nettelbladt and Håkansson, 1991). Apart from syntax, Swedish morphology also causes problems to the learner, in particular verb morphology (i.e. finiteness and tense) and the morphology of the noun (i.e. number, gender and definiteness).

Phonologically, the consonant system is almost as complicated as that of English, and, in particular, non-labial fricatives and liquids cause children problems. The vowel system includes front, rounded vowels, which are acquired late. What makes Swedish, together with Norwegian, sound somewhat exotic, however, is the relatively complicated prosodic system. There are both contrasts of stress, i.e. initial versus non-initial stress, and of tonal accent, i.e. accent 1 and accent 2. Stress and tonal accent are thus different categories as shown by the following triplet: Càllas (name), 'kallas (called), ka'la:s (party) (for further details, see Nettelbladt, 1983). Within a sentence or textual perspective, there is an intricate relationship between the phonetic realisation of tonal accents of the individual words, placement of sentence accent and its relation to position within the utterance (Bruce, 1977). The phonetic realisation of the word accents varies across different regional dialects in Sweden and word and sentence accents are salient characteristics of a person's regional identity. One of the more prominent problems in children with severe language impairment concerns the development of tonal accents and of sentence prosody, and, as a consequence, these children often lack a clear prosodic identity (Nettlebladt, 1983: Nettlebladt et al., 1989).

This article will focus on multidisciplinary research on children with specific but severe language impairment carried out at Lund University Hospital during the last 8 years. The starting point of our research has been, and still is, clinical. My own direction of research could mainly be characterised as clinical linguistics, very much following the tradition from Great Britain. Working within a multidisciplinary framework has forced me to define the analytical tools more carefully. It has also called for revisions of the traditional, linguistic descriptive methods. Another reason for the successive revisions of our descriptive tools lies in the data itself: when you gradually get more and more into the language of these enigmatic children new, previously unknown phenomena of language suddenly appear. These data may not fit into the descriptive models at hand and you are left with the decision to either ignore these data or to revise your models. As this chapter will show, we have chosen the latter alternative.

The chapter reviews the research leading up to where we stand today. It is organised around three successive but interrelated studies. The three studies involve different groups of children, with ten subjects within each study. In all three studies a case study approach has been applied. The reason for choosing such an approach was that, from the outset, we knew very little of the characteristics of language impairment in Swedish children. We thus needed to pinpoint each individual child's language in order to achieve an in-depth analysis of the child's language impairment. Our focus on qualitatively based case studies does not, however, preclude quantification.

### Study 1: Subgroups of Phonological Impairment

The first is a longitudinal study on phonological disorders in children with language impairment.The research, compiled in my doctoral thesis (Nettelbladt, 1983) was restricted to phonological aspects of language, and was not multidisciplinary. The analytic framework presented in the thesis mirrored trends in child phonology research in the early 1980s, in particular work by Menn (1978) and Waterson (1971). It also stemmed from reorientations in general phonology, viz. Metric Phonology (Hayes, 1981; Selkirk, 1981), where the prosodic organisation of words and phrases is taken into account.

Ten children with different degrees of language disorder were studied longitudinally for 2–3 years in late preschool age to after entry into school (children do not begin school in Sweden until age 7). The main finding was that the children differed not only with regard to the amount of phonological simplifications involved but also with respect to the types of simplifications. Five of the children, who were assessed by their clinicians as having a severe language impairment, showed syntagmatic restrictions, i.e. a simplified word and syllable structure with deletions of unstressed syllables, deletions of consonant clusters, deletions of word-final consonants resulting in open CV-syllables. They also showed reduplications and assimilations. Further, they were aberrant in their prosodic development, since they lacked contrasts of stress and accent. In addition, they had paradigmatic processes, i.e. context-free consonant and vowel substitutions.

The other five children, assessed as having a less severe or moderate language impairment, showed paradigmatic processes only, restricted to

**Table 11.1.** Productions with syntagmatic and paradigmatic restriction

| Target | Syntagmatic production | Paradigmatic production |
|---|---|---|
| ambu 'lans ('ambulance') | ba: | abuð' a:t |
| ɛ:ɪəR ('eats') | 'ta:ta: | 'ɛ :ɪə |
| 'nɛ :san ('the nose') | 'sa:sa: | 'nɛ :tan |

consonants. Table 11.1 illustrates productions with syntagmatic and paradigmatic restrictions respectively.

A concomitant finding was that all the children with syntagmatic restrictions had a grammatical disability. This was not found in the children with only paradigmatic processes, who were either normally developed grammatically or had only traces of earlier grammatical problems. It seemed likely that the syntagmatic restrictions within the children's phonology and their grammatical problems were interrelated. Problems with hierarchical organisation, a concept described by Cromer (1981), was suggested as a common denominator.

The most important finding of Study 1 was that the children with syntagmatic restrictions did not only have a more severe and generalised language impairment in comparison with the children with only paradigmatic restrictions. A syntagmatically based phonological disorder appeared to be qualitatively different or deviant in contrast to a paradigmatically based disorder, which could be considered as a phonological delay. The reader is reminded of the debate on deviance and delay in language disorders, (cf. Ingram, 1976; Leonard, 1980), a debate which seems to have come to a standstill, (though see Grimm and Weinert (1990)). Although Study 1 was purely linguistic, the results initiated the multidisciplinary approach applied in later studies.

### Study 2: A Cross-sectional Study of Ten Children with Severe Language Impairment

The results from the first study indicated that the children with laguage impairment constituted a heterogeneous group with respect to aetiology, underlying neuropsychological dysfunctions and linguistic symptoms. A widening of research perspectives was necessary, not only linguistically (see Hansson, 1991; Hansson and Nettelbladt, 1990, 1991), but also beyond discipline boundaries.

In order to plan for the next study, a research team was established with representatives from different clinical disciplines: clinical linguistics, aphasiology and neurolinguistics, neuropaediatrics and child psychology. A detailed description of the methodology used and the results is given in Nettelbladt et al. (1989).

With the aim of testing out possible diagnostic methods, an extensive array of procedures was applied. The neurolinguistic assessments aimed at relating different neuropsychological functions to thorough linguistic descriptions of the children's communicative behaviour. The assessment used is called NELLI, a neurolinguistic examination procedure for children with language disorders (Holmberg and Sahlén, 1986), which is founded on Luria's neuropsychological theory and principles for investigation. It involves a number of different tasks, for example, tactile and kinaesthetic tasks, visual and visuospatial tasks, motor and oral motor tasks, non-verbal and verbal auditory tasks, phoneme discrimination, word mobilisation and description of thematic pictures. The NELLI is not standardised but all the different tasks have been administered to groups of normal children of varying ages in order to obtain age-references.

The children were video and audio taped during the assessment, during which was elicited spontaneous speech. Parts of the extensive taped material were transcribed phonetically and orthographically by two independent transcribers. Subsequent comparisons of the transcriptions showed substantial agreement; discrepancies were either resolved by joint listening or dismissed. The linguistic analyses were based on the transcribed material and focused on phonology and grammar. The reader is referred to Nettelbladt (1983) and Hansson and Nettelbladt (1990), for details regarding the phonological and grammatical analyses. For the psychological examination, the children were tested with the Griffith Mental Developmental Scale, and the two oldest children with the WISC. The study also included a qualitative assessment of the child's behaviour and a parental interview.

The medical assessment included a careful neuropaediatric examination, an assessment by a physiotherapist and a number of medical examinations, for example computed tomography of the brain, analysis of the spinal fluid, chromosome analysis, neurometabolic screenings and EEG recordings. In addition, the child underwent a thorough audiological evaluation.

Ten children, who were referred for assessment because of a severe language impairment, served as subjects. There were eight boys and two girls within quite a large age span: 4–10 years. An important factor in selecting the children was that their parents were willing to let their child participate in the extensive examinations required.

The results revealed few links between medical findings and findings in other areas. The psychological assessment revealed that some of the children used a dysfunctional strategy in coping with their handicap, which in some cases appeared to conceal the child's basic problem. A general finding was that, at times, different results were arrived at, although the subtests and tasks used (for example the Griffith, the physiotherapist's testing and the NELLI), were meant to assess the same function in the child. The results from the neurolinguistic examination revealed the following profiles: three children had problems predominantly within the verbal-auditory domain, two children had mainly motor problems. The remaining five children had combinations of perceptuomotor and attentional problems.

The linguistic analyses showed some features we might tentatively connect with the neurolinguistic profiles. Two of the children with auditory problems used phonological rules inconsistently, whereas one child with motor and visuospatial problems used systematic, rigid rules. Grammatically, the two children with auditory problems had a tendency to duplicate words which made their utterances appear longer and structurally more complex than they were. Their relatively normal sentence prosody appeared to serve as a compensatory means to give this impression. With the remaining children no such connections were found.

We also compared our findings with currently used classification systems for children with language disorders, viz. the systems described by Rapin and Allen (1983, 1987) and by Bishop and Rosenbloom (1987). Most of the children in the study could best be classified as belonging to the phonological–syntactic subtype. One of the children was classified as semantic–pragmatic and one child, who was extremely difficult to test, showed some autistic traits and was later diagnosed as mentally retarded. In fact, all the children who had combinations of perceptuomotor and attentional problems were found to have more general problems and were less specifically language impaired. They were also among the older children within the group.

As earlier mentioned, there were few links between the medical and the other examinations. However, in later years new techniques within computer technology are being developed at the Department of Neurophysiology at Lund University Hospital. Brain mapping enables a topographical analysis of electrophysiological brain activity. Preliminary results from a pilot study give some evidence of regional differences in the electrophysiological brain acitivty in disordered children as compared to normal controls (Ors et al., 1992).

## Study 3: A Longitudinal Study of Ten Children with Severe Language Disorder

In order to explore further the possibilities of finding connections between the neurolinguistic profiles and the linguistic characteristics, a longitudinal study was initiated in cooperation with Birgitta Sahlén. Ten children with severe language disorders were selected from the first generations of children to attend the newly started language preschool unit in Lund. The subjects were seven boys and three girls. They were quite homogeneous with respect to age. The recordings started when the children had recently started preschool, at approximately 4 years of age. Recordings have been made at least yearly until 8 years.

Since the connections between the linguistic and the neurolinguistic analyses from Study 2 appeared most promising we decided to concentrate on these two kinds of analyses. The neurolinguistic examination was identical to that employed in the earlier study. The linguistic analyses were supplemented with a more detailed interaction analysis (Linell, Gustavsson and Juvonen, 1988; Hansson and Nettelbladt, 1990; Nettelbladt and Hansson, 1991). The interaction analysis proved especially helpful in analyzing the dialogues with children with semantic-pragmatic problems (see the last section of this chapter and Sahlén, Nettelbladt and Dravins, 1991).

The results from Study 3 are quite extensive and only a summary of the most important findings is given here. The reader is referred to several articles (Sahlén, Wigforss and Nettelbladt, 1990; Sahlén et al., 1991; Sahlén and Löfqvist, 1991; Sahlén and Nettelbladt, 1991a; Sahlén and Nettelbladt, 1991b).

The neurolinguistic examination revealed two gross subgroups of dysfunctions: auditory problems and motor problems; only two of the children had additional visuospatial problems. As Table 11.2 shows, the phonological–syntactic subtype was by far the most common: seven children out of the ten were considered phonological–syntactic. One child was assessed as lexical–syntactic. The remaining two children, both of which are girls, were considered semantic–pragmatic.

The neurolinguistic profiles of the children were as follows: six children had problems predominantly within the auditory domain. (Auditory functions were assessed with the following tasks: phoneme discrimination; language comprehension, e.g. logic–grammatical constructions; verbal auditory productive tasks, i.e. different repetition tasks as, for example, repetition of lists of semantically unrelated words and retelling a story; repetition of sentences and sequences of nonsense syllables.)

Three of the children had problems predominantly within the motor domain. (Motor functions were assessed with the following tasks: oral motor tasks, either isolated or within a dynamic sequence; word mobilisation, i.e. timed retrieval of words in a given semantic category; nonverbal and verbal repetition tasks, i.e. sequences of rhythm and of nonsense syllables and verbal praxis, e.g. repetition of syllables, nonsense

**Table 11.2.** Classification of the children in Study 3

| Child | Phonological– syntactic | Lexical– syntactic | Semantic– pragmatic |
|-------|-------------------------|--------------------|---------------------|
| Jarl | X (M) | | |
| Albert | X (M) | | |
| Mns | X (M) | | |
| Julia | X (A) | | |
| Jesper | X (A) | | |
| Oskar | X (A) | | |
| Knut | X (A) | | |
| Jonas | | X (A) | |
| Marta | | | X (A) |
| Lena | | | X (A) |
| Total | (7) | (1) | (2) |

M = Motor problems; A = Auditory problems.

words and tongue-twister words; confrontation naming. During testing, the phonological problems of the child were taken into consideration.)

Within each of these two groups there was considerable variation in terms of degree of impairment and also regarding which level or levels were affected. Some of the children were relatively mildly affected, for example had problems restricted to phoneme discrimination and repetition of tongue-twister words, whereas other children had more generalised problems within language comprehension: tasks involving lexical categorisation and retellling of a story.

Since the longitudinal framework permitted us to study the children for an extensive time span, we gradually became interested in prognostic factors (cf. Bishop and Edmundson, 1987). First, it is obvious that all the children were much more globally impaired at 4 and also at 5 years but gradually their symptoms became more circumscribed. Secondly, the children with severe comprehension problems, with a poor lexical-semantic and semantic-pragmatic development are much more at risk for persisting language problems than children with less global problems.This is in spite of the fact that the children with poorer prognosis had relatively mild phonological and grammatical problems. Thirdly, the children with persisting phonological problems had oral motor problems in combination with a delayed motor development in general.

When trying to characterise the children linguistically in greater detail, it was found that both the phonological and the grammatical analyses needed revision.

## Phonological Analysis Reconsidered

It was an interesting but frustrating finding that all the children within the phonological–syntactic group showed basically the same types of phonological simplifications, especially in terms of consonant substitutions. But many of the syntagmatic restrictions were also similar across the children, including problems with prosodic contrasts. To a large extent, they also had the same kind of grammatical problems, e.g. problems with omissions of function words and of bound morphemes and problems with word order in topicalised sentences and placement of negation. This was in spite of the fact that they had different neurolinguistic profiles and that some of these children did sound differently both phonologically and grammatically.

Accordingly, we went back to the tapes, retranscribed parts of the material, and, most important, we asked two independent listeners, both trained phoneticians, to assess some of the material. Up to now, five children from the longitudinal study have been assessed. We selected recordings from later ages; 6 and 8 years, since the problems at these ages were less global. We also believed that these ages were more representative of the individual child's neurolinguistic profile. The results are tentative and have to be tried out on more data and, preferably, be presented to larger groups of professional listeners.

On the basis of our findings so far, we will suggest modifications of our traditional phonological analysis as follows. The dynamics of speech production has to be captured, in particular, speech rate: it was found to be much slower in children with motor problems than in children with basically auditory problems. In a recent study, Sahlén and Löfqvist (1991) found significant differences with respect to rate of repetition of nonsense syllables in two of the children in the phonological–syntactic group, one considered auditorily defective, the other with motor problems.

Related to the slow speech rate was an impression of staccato rhythmic patterns, which we believe is due to a more basic lack of rhythmic alternation, i.e. alternation between stressed and unstressed syllables, typical of natural fast speech (Bruce, 1987). Lack of rhythmic alternation influences sentence intonation which gets smoothed down, very much due to the slow rate.

Thus, we need to describe larger domains of speech, not only the phonology of segments and words. For example, problems with word accents do not appear to be such a critical differentiating symptom as we believed in the first and the second studies. These findings have led us to question the traditional division of linguistic levels and, in particular the overemphasis on segmental phonology in clinical linguistics. Prosody appears to be an important link between phonology and grammar, and, possibly also to semantics. Our findings and focus on prosody can partly be attributed to the fact that Swedish has quite an intricate prosodic system.

## Extensions of the Grammatical Analysis

Another frustration with regard to the linguistic analyses was that is was hard to find other but quite subtle phonological and grammatical problems in the children referred to as semantic–pragmatic. In particular, some grammatical subtleties did not appear to be captured by our analyses. We found that these children superficially sounded prosodically normal. (This was similar to the findings in Study 2 of the two children with auditory problems but who belonged to the phonological–syntactic group.) The two children with semantic–pragmatic disorder had a normal speech rate and they did alternate their speech rhythm. At a first glance it even seemed as if they used quite adequate syntactic structures

A reanalysis of transcripts based on a more comprehensive representation of the whole discourse, rather than treating single sentences separately, revealed the following. The grammatical repertoire of the two children was limited but with few grammatical errors. The normal grammatical patterns often consisted of phrases that were repeated over and over again, which gave a stereotypical impression with recurring, also stereotypical prosodic patterns. Insertions of dummy syllables and of dummy words were quite frequent. Our auditory assessments also revealed that the vocal behaviour of the two semantic–pragmatic children was aberrant. Hesitation phenomena were also very prominent in one of the two children who had more extensive grammatical problems from the beginning. Semantically related grammatical errors occurred as well. The suggested extension of grammatical analysis is related to recent work by Miller (1987) and Fletcher (1987). A study reported on in Hansson (1991) and Hansson and Nettelbladt (1991) found that children with a grammatical impairment used a significantly larger amount of hesitation than children with a phonological impairment only.

## Towards an Interactionally and Contextually Differentiated Pragmatic Assessment

In conclusion, a brief excursion will be made to a separate study made on the two children with semantic-pragmatic disorders (Sahlén et al., 1991). For the analysis of their communicative behaviour the so-called initiative–response analysis was used (Linell, Gustavsson and Juvonen, 1988). Rather than categorising individual utterances as speech acts, it is interactionally based, i.e. it takes into account local, sequential properties, the retroactive and proactive links of turns. Although this analysis is concerned with coding and quantitative measures, it has certain features in common with conversational analysis as developed within ethnomethodology (Heritage, 1984). The interaction analysis used focuses upon the interactional cooperation between each participant and the gradual development of the dialogue. The analysis has been used within another research project where children with language impairment are studied together with different conversational partners (Nettelbladt and Hansson, 1991).

The interaction analysis of the two children with semantic–pragmatic disorder (Sahlén et al., 1991) showed a close resemblance to the findings of other studies on children with semantic–pragmatic disorder with regard to deviant communicative behaviour (e.g. Adams and Bishop, 1989; Bishop and Adams, 1989; Conti-Ramsden and Gunn, 1986). Such deviant patterns were conspicous lack of responses, fragmentary or tangential responses and abrupt topic shifts without any summons. Obviously, finding such types of deviant patterns are important for diagnostic purposes, to demarcate children with semantic–pragmatic disorders from other types of language impairment.

However, the interaction analysis also revealed some unexpected patterns of interaction, which appear to be more relevant for their therapeutic potentials. Interspersed within the deviant parts of the dialogues were sequences of perfectly normal, fluent and reciprocal interaction. When scrutinising these sequences it was found that they occurred under specific conditions: when the child was initiating the conversation, selected the topic or when the topic was familiar to the child. These normal sequences were not found when the child was asked direct questions or other demands were put to the child. Our interpretation of these findings is that the child's comprehension was not hampered or distracted during these normal sequences, in other words, children with pragmatic problems may function much more normally than assumed but only under optimal conditions.

An interaction analysis such as the one used in Sahlén et al. (1991) appears to be a fruitful tool to provide us with insights for therapy. Knowledge of the healthy aspects of the child's behaviour may be obscured using pragmatic assessments with a fault-finding focus on aberrant behaviour. An interactional approach could be further explored clinically by studying the same child across varying contextual demands and with different conversational partners (Fey and Leonard, 1983; Nettelbladt and Hansson, 1991).

## Acknowledgements

Paul Fletcher and my colleagues at Lund University are thanked for their helpful comments on earlier drafts of the manuscript. The research reported on in this chapter has been supported in parts by grants from Lund University, grants nos. 86/73, 86/105 and 90/211 from Bank of Sweden Tercentenary Foundation and a grant from the Foundation of Sävstaholm.

## References

ADAMS, C. and BISHOP, D. (1989). Conversational characteristics of children with semantic-pragmatic disorder. I. Exchange structure, turntaking, repairs and cohesion. *British Journal of Disorders of Communication*, 24, 211–239.

BISHOP, D. and ADAMS, C. (1989). Conversational characteristics of children with semantic-pragmatic disorder. II. What features lead to a judgment of inappropriacy? *British Journal of Disorders of Communication*, 24, 241–263.

BISHOP, D. and EDMUNDSON, A (1987). Language-impaired 4 year olds: Distinguishing transient from persistent impairment. *Journal of Speech and Hearing Disorders*, 52, 156–173.

BISHOP, D. and ROSENBLOOM, L. (1987). Childhood language disorders: classification and overview. In: Yule, W. and Rutter, M. (Eds.), *Language Development and Disorders. Clinics in Developmental Medicine, 101/102*, pp. 16–41. London: Mac-Keith Press.

BRUCE, G. (1977). *Swedish Word Accents in Sentence Perspective*. Lund: Gleerup.

BRUCE, G. (1987). On the phonology and phonetics of rhythm: Evidence from Swedish. *Proceedings of the Fifth International Phonology Meeting, Eisenstadt, June, 1984. Phonologica, 1984*, pp. 21–31. Cambridge: CUP

CONTI-RAMSDEN, G. and GUNN, M. (1986). The development of conversational disability: a case study. *British Journal of Disorders of Communication*, 21, 339–352.

CROMER, R. (1981). Hierarchical ordering disability and aphasic children. In: Dale, P. and Ingram, D. (Eds), *Child Language: An International Perspective*, pp. 319–330. Baltimore: University Park Press.

FEY, M. and LEONARD, L. (1983). Pragmatic skills of children with specific language impairment. In: Gallagher, T. and Prutting, C. (Eds), *Pragmatic Assessment and Intervention Issues in Language*, pp. 65–82. San Diego: College-Hill Press.

FLETCHER, P. (1987). The basis of language impairment in children: a comment on Chiat and Hirson. *British Journal of Disorders of Communication*, 22, 65–72.

GRIMM, H. and WEINERT, S. (1990). Is the syntax development of dysphasic children deviant and why? *Journal of Speech and Hearing Research*, 33, 220–228.

HANSSON, K. (1991). Aspects of grammatical disorder in Swedish preschool children. Paper presented at the Second International Symposium on Specific Speech and Language Disorders in Children, Harrogate, 26–30 May, 1991.

HANSSON, K. and NETTELBLADT, U. (1990). The verbal interaction of Swedish language disordered preschool children. *Clinical Linguistics and Phonetics*, 4, 39–48.

HANSSON, K. and NETTELBLADT, U (1991). Swedish children with dysgrammatism. A comparison with normally developed children. *Working Papers in Logopedics and Phoniatrics*, 7. Lund: Lund University.

HAYES, B (1981). *A Metrical Theory of Stress Rules*. Bloomington: Indiana University Linguistics Club.

HOLMBERG, E and SAHLÉN, B. (1986). *NELLI - Neurolingvistisk undersökningsmodell för språkstörda barn*. Malmö:Utbildningsproduktion AB.

HÅKANSSON, G. (1988). Hungry I am – breakfast I want. On the acquisition of inverted word order in Swedish. *Working Papers*, 33, 123–130, Department of Linguistics, Lund University.

HYLTENSTAM, K. (1977). Implicational patterns in interlanguage syntax variation. *Language Learning*, 27, 383–411.

HERITAGE, J. (1984). *Garfinkel and Ethnomethodology*. Cambridge and Oxford: Polity Press.

INGRAM, D. (1976). *Phonological Disability in Children*. London: Edward Arnold.

LEONARD, L. (1980). The speech of language-disabled children. *Bulletin of the Orton Society*, 30, 141–152.

LEONARD, L., SABBADINI, L., LEONARD, J. and VOLTERRA, V. (1987). Specific language impairment in children: a cross-linguistic study. *Brain and Language*, 32, 233–252.

LINELL, P., GUSTAVSSON, L. and JUVONEN, P. (1988). Interactional dominance in dyadic communication: a presentation of initiative–response analysis. *Linguistics*, 26, 415–442.

MILLER, J. (1987). A grammatical characterization of language disorder. In: Martin, A. Fletcher, P.,Grunwell, P. and Hall, D. (Eds), *Proceedings of the First International Symposium on Specific Speech and Language Disorders in Children*, pp. 100–113. Reading: University of Reading.

MENN, L. (1978). *Pattern, Control and Contrast in Beginning Speech. A Case Study in the Development of Word Form and Word Function*. Bloomington: Indiana University Linguistics Club.

NETTELBLADT, U. (1983). *Developmental Studies of Dysphonology in Children*. Lund: Liber.

NETTELBLADT, U. and HANSSON, K. (1991). Dialogues with language disordered children. How does the interactional style of the conversational partner influence the child? In: Mjaavatn, P., Hagtvedt, B. and Feilberg, J. (Eds), *Proceedings From the 2nd Meeting of the European Group for Child Language Disorders*, Røros, Norway, 1990. The Norwegian Centre for Child Research, Report no. 24, 137–148.

NETTELBLADT, U. and HÅKANSSON, G. (1992). Towards an integrated view on language acquisition. Could work with language disordered children profit from theories of first and second language acquisition? *Scandinavian Journal of Logopedics and Phoniatrics*, 1 (in press).

NETTELBLADT, U., SAHLÉN, B., ORS, M. and JOHANNESSON, P. (1989). A multidisciplinary assessment of chidren with severe language disorder. *Clinical Linguistics and Phonetics*, 3, 313–346.

ORS, M., STENBERG, G., ROSÉN, I, MAGNUSSON, C., SAHLÉN, B., LÖFQVIST, A., NETTELBLADT, U. and BLENNOW, G. (1992) *Topographic Analysis of Electrophysiological Brain Activity in Children with Specific Language Impairment*. Lund: Departments of Neurophysiology, Pediatrics and Logopedics and Phoniatrics, Lund University Hospital.

RAPIN, L. and ALLEN, D. A. (1983). Developmental language disorders. Nosologic considerations. In: Kirk, U. (Ed.), *Neuropsychology of Language, Reading and Spelling*, pp. 155–183. New York: Academic Press.

RAPIN, I. and ALLEN, D. A. (1987). Developmental dysphasia and autism in preschool children: Characteristics and subtypes. In: Martin, A,. Fletcher, P.,Grunwell, P. and Hall, D. (Eds), *Proceedings of the First International Symposium on Specific Speech and Language Disorders in Children*, pp. 20–35. Reading: University of Reading.

SAHLÉN, B. and LÖFQVIST, A. (1991). Linguistic and dynamic modes of description of developmental language disorders. In: Sahlén, B. (ed.), *From Depth to Surface. A Case Study Approach to Severe Development Language Disorders*. Lund: Studentlitteratur.

SAHLÉN, B. and NETTELBLADT, U. (1991a). Patterns of vulnerability of language in children with severe developmental language disorders. In: Sahlén, B. (Ed.), *From Depth to Surface. A Case Study Approach to Severe Development Language Disorders.* Lund: Studentlitteratur.

SAHLÉN, B, and NETTELBLADT, U. (1991b). A longitudinal study of ten children with severe developmental language disorders. In: Sahlén, B. (Ed.), *From Depth to Surface. A Case Study Approach to Severe Development Language Disorders.* Lund: Studentlitteratur.

SAHLÉN, B., NETTELBLADT, U. and DRAVINS, C. (1991). Children with semantic-pragmatic disorder and posterior aphasics – what do they have in common? In: Sahlén, B. (Ed.), *From Depth to Surface. A Case Study Approach to Severe Development Language Disorders.* Lund: Studentlitteratur.

SAHLÉN, B., WIGFORSS, E. and NETTELBLADT, U. (1990). Severe developmental language disorder – reading and spelling. A longitudinal study of two non-identical twins. *Reading and Writing: An Interdisciplinary Journal,* 2, 269–295.

SELKIRK, E. (1981). On prosodic structure and its relation to syntactic structure. In Fretheim, T (Ed.). *Nordic Prosody II,* pp. 111–140. Trondheim: Tapir Press.

WATERSON, N. (1971). Child phonology: a prosodic view. *Journal of Linguistics,* 7, 179–211.

# Chapter 12
# Sub-groups in school-age language-impaired children

PAUL FLETCHER

## Introduction

The first AFASIC symposium was rich in information and ideas. Because of resonances with my own work at the time, I was particularly struck by Jon Miller's paper on the grammatical characterisation of language disorder, in which he discussed a clinically derived typology of language disorders in school-age children. He suggested in his paper that 'clinicians know from their clinical experience that there are several types of language disorder in children', and that this clinical intuition required some detailed research investigation. 'Variation reported in language performance, particularly among older language-disordered children, suggests serious consideration must be given to sub-groups of disorders defined by distinct language performance'. The range of disorder types that Miller had in mind, as illustrated in his paper, appears in Figure 12.1. While, as Miller pointed out, none of these terms was new, there are two significant points to be made about the list. First, the terms were intended to represent a taxonomy of deficits across which the disordered population might be distributed. And second, the hypothesis that these were independent language deficits had to be tested against extensive samples of their output language performance.

For the idea that subtypes of disorder existed was not new. At the time of the first symposium in 1987 a fairly extensive literature on the typology of language impairment was available (see, e.g. Aram and Nation, 1975; Wolfus, Moscovitch and Kinsbourne 1980; Wren, 1980; Rapin, 1982; Crystal, 1986; Risucci and Wilson, 1986). There are three broad groups into which the studies then extant can be divided, which we can refer to as clinical, psychometric and linguistic.

1.      Sentence formulation problems

2.      Word-finding problems

3.      Rate and fluency problems

4.      Hyperverbosity

5.      Pragmatic/discourse problems

6.      Semantic and referencing deficits

**Figure 12.1** Categories of language disorder (from Miller 1989).

The best-known of the clinical subtyping procedures was that provided by Rapin and her associates (e.g. Rapin, 1982; Rapin and Allen, 1982). This is an approach which relies on a clinical syndrome of identification of clusters of behaviours observed across a large number of individuals. The Rapin/Allen classification identified six subgroups of children with developmental language disability. While the groupings may seem to fit with our experience (e.g. phonological programming deficit for developmental verbal dyspraxia), they are perhaps at too great a level of abstraction (e.g. phonological/syntactic syndrome), to link easily with Miller's proposed categories. The psychometric approach attempts to classify children with language impairment using multivariate statistical procedures on the children's performance on a battery of standardised tests. A project of particular interest is that of Wilson and Risucci (1986) which attempts to validate statistically a clinically derived subgrouping. While their classification works well in terms of its external validation, the majority of tests (or subtests) included in the battery do not directly address linguistic competence. There does not appear to be, within the 30 measurement procedures used, a single measure of expressive syntax, for example. The tests were selected to measure factors thought to be relevant to language disability (e.g. auditory perception, auditory memory, visual memory) and language production performance was not directly addressed.

There are, however, two linguistic studies which are perhaps more in the spirit of the enquiry Miller is encouraging. Wren (1980) used measures derived from LARSP syntactic profiles (Crystal, Fletcher and Garman, 1989) to try to identify types of disorder in a group of 30 'language learning disabled children' between 6 and 7 years of age. She used a factor analysis which yielded two identifiable subgroups. At least one of these appears to be comparable to the category Miller calls 'sentence formulation problems'. The second study of interest, by Crystal (1986), also involved an analysis of 30 children, this time over a more disparate age range, from just under 5 years to just over 10 years. Crystal also used

LARSP syntactic variables, but in addition included semantic and non-fluency measures. In a cluster analysis of this data, one clear group that emerges may relate to either Miller's category 2 – word-finding problems, or to his category 3 – rate and fluency problems.

A satisfactory typology of language disorders in school-age children would presumably have features of all three of these approaches. It should provide clinically valid sub-groups. It should, ultimately, be psychometrically adequate. Also, if it is the case that a language-impaired population exists as (in Wilson and Risucci's (1986) words) 'a relatively discrete class of neurologically based disorders', it ought to be possible to characterise this in terms of their linguistic behaviour, provided a suitable model for that behaviour is available. It would also be advantageous if the approach to sub-classification permitted subtyping in terms of a multidimensional profile, rather than attempting to fix children within clear-cut, mutually exclusive categories (Bishop, 1989).

### The Data and the Model

My purpose in this paper is to re-analyse the Crystal (1986) data within a multidimensional profile in order to try to identify subtypes of language output performance behaviour. First, however, I need to justify the use of output performance data, the model within which these data are to be interpreted, and the relationship between the analysis categories and the model.

*Data.* A few words in favour of what is known as spontaneous speech data may be relevant at this point. From one point of view language production has the irritating quality of being largely under the control of the speaker rather than the investigator. The speaker may choose to respond or not to a particular stimulus, and ultimately decides on the syntax and lexis appropriate for the intended message. So for hypothesis testing, or even reliable description, it might appear that spontaneous speech data has serious disadvantages. A skilled interlocutor is not without influence however (as speech therapists are well aware) and ingenious contextual manipulation can often virtually dictate quite specific syntactic structures (as demonstrated for example by Crain, NcKee and Emiliani, 1990 for the elicitation of relative clauses). Second, extensive stretches of speech can reveal distinct patterns of strength and weakness in various aspects of linguistic competence – the grammatical system, the prosodic system, lexis. The third argument one might deploy in favour of databases of spontaneous speech is that, properly transcribed to include pauses, mazes and other fluency characteristics, they provide us with evidence of the language production processing system in operation. Which brings us to the model.

*The Model.* It seems unlikely that a perspective on language production behaviour which involves grammatical and lexical categories only will be enough. Miller's clinical types involve word-finding and fluency, and Crystal has already identified non-fluency as a salient variable in his analysis. These are not syntactic categories as generally recognised via a LARSP or similar profile. We also know from other studies that comparisons between school-age normal and language-impaired children, in terms of their representational ability – the linguistic structures of which they appear to have command – show up very limited differences. To quote from a recent paper by Curtis and Tallal (1991) 'LI children appear to be constructing the same grammars, in the same way, as normal children.' While this is perhaps, in our present state of knowledge, a somewhat sweeping conclusion, it is a view that has some merit. While the timescale may be very different, the structures available to LI children look very like those available to normals. The differences between them and normals seem to lie in the LI children's ability to *deploy* these structural resources under the real-time demands of conversation. If we want to consider not only what syntactic resources are available to the speaker, but how these resources are deployed in real time, it seems we need to broaden our perspective on what aspect of the speaker's linguistic knowledge we address. We should consider speaking not just in terms of its product – a set of syntactic structures – but as a production system which gets from 'conceptual intention to utterance' (Chiat and Hirson, 1987) in real time. Clearly syntactic structures are a central part of the language production system. But in the data from which we extract the syntactic structure categories – samples of the child's speech – there is a wealth of other information, naturally displayed, of the language production system in action.

Figure 12. 2 represents schematically an outline of the language production system as a blueprint for the speaker – as constructed by Levelt (1989). It is sentence-based: it assumes that the messages a speaker encodes will be essentially propositional in nature. It is dynamic: it involves (in either series or parallel) structure-building appropriate for the message in both grammatical and phonological codes, using available lexical information; and it is subject to continuous monitoring, on-line, the effects of which may show up at any point in the utterance being articulated. The speed with which all this has to happen is quite staggering on reflection (Lieberman, 1991 estimates that we produce between 25 and 50 words per second) and it is not surprising that some individuals may be more or less efficient than others.

Figure 12.2 represents then an account of the architecture of a complex processing system, which is conceived of as independent of, though of course in various ways it must be linked to, other cognitive systems. In addition (as Levelt, 1989 makes clear) each component within the

1. **Conceptualiser**
   Encodes a pre-verbal message as input to formulator. Monitors speaker's own speech.

2. **Formulator**
   **(A) Grammatical Encoder**
   > i)Accesses lemmas from lexicon appropriate for message.
   > ii)Builds syntactic structures for lexical items.

   **(B) Phonological Encoder**
   Provides phonological form and builds a phonetic or articulatory plan for each lexical item and for the utterance as a whole.

   **(C) Articulator**
   Implements the articulatory plan.

**Figure 12.2** A blueprint for the speaker (after Levelt 1989).

system is viewed as relatively autonomous, a specialist in its own work. So the grammatical encoder is, for example, a specialist in translating a pre-verbal message into grammatical relations. There is no other part of the system that is able to do this. Similarly only the phonological encoder can provide the lexical item GIVE, say, with its characteristic phonological form.

If this view of the language production process is valid, then the potential exists for it to operate less than efficiently. We know that the system operates at less than optimum efficiency for normal adults on occasion. Indeed, slips of the tongue on the part of normal speakers constitute part of the evidence used for the type of model outlined in Figure 12.2. Such errors are relatively rare in normals, however. It would be possible, presumably, for an impaired individual's system to be considerably less efficient, and for a wider range of errors to occur, at various stages of the operating system. If we could identify and locate the errors in terms of the operating system, and in particular identify different classes of error, we might be able to argue for sub-types of impairment in a principled way.

In a detailed case study which used a language production process perspective, Chiat and Hirson (1987) were successful in identifying one type of problem. Their subject's expressive difficulties looked bewilderingly various if described within a syntactic profile. However, if the responsibility for these problems was assigned to the *phonological encoding* stage of the production model, a consistent explanation was possible. The child seemed to have other components of the model intact, but had difficulty processing detail within a rhythmic structure, which led to the omission of unstressed syllables, particularly, sometimes in quite lengthy syntactic strings.

Chiat and Hirson (1987) suggested that the problem they had analysed was a quite general one. It seems unlikely, however, that all school-age language impairment reduces to phonological problems quite late in the production process. To test this requires a group of subjects, and categories of analysis which would connect to the proposed model and yet be general enough to show up any patterns in the data. In a study of 15 school-age language-impaired children first reported in 1989, we used six analysis categories, relating to fluency, to grammatical competence, and to types of errors. There were two types of error we were particularly interested in: those that, like Chiat and Hirson's, could be plausibly attributed to the phonological encoder; and those which we could locate in the grammatical encoder. The results were interesting. Of the 15 subjects 9 fell clearly, in terms of their profiles on the categories of analysis used, into four groups. The groups and their salient characteristics are listed in Table 12.1.

**Table 12.1** Subtypes of language production impairments (from Fletcher, 1991)

|         | Fluency | Grammar | Grerr | Pherr |
|---------|---------|---------|-------|-------|
| Group 1 | Good    | Hi      | Lo    | Lo    |
| Group 2 | Poor    | Lo      | Hi    | Hi    |
| Group 3 | Poor    | Hi      | Hi    | Lo    |
| Group 4 | Poor    | Mod     | Hi    | Lo    |

An informative comparison here can be made between Groups 1 and 2, each comprising two boys. The performance of Group 2 on the categories of the profile is the exact complement of Group 1. Group 2 is relatively disfluent, has relatively poor grammatical structure building capacity, and has a high proportion of errors of both types. Group 1 does not have fluency problems, has adequate structure-building ability, and does not make many errors in production. We might claim, on this basis, that in fact Group 1 has, relative to the status of their representational linguistic system, no obvious production processing problems, and the basis for their clinical diagnosis as language-impaired must lie elsewhere. In Miller's terms, we would want to investigate pragmatic/discourse problems, and semantic/referencing deficits. Group 2, on the other hand, show difficulties at various levels of the model in the deployment of their linguistic knowledge. Groups 3 and 4 (three and two children respectively) can also be interpreted within the language production model. They are of interest by comparison with Group 2 because they show that it is possible to have distinct difficulties with grammatical and phonological encoding. All these children seem to produce more errors at the grammatical encoding stage than the phonological.

The first attempt to look at group data in terms of a multidimensional profile whose categories were linked to a language production model thus seemed promising. The categories appeared to be independent of one another (in fact there were no significant inter-correlations between the categories used). The approach also seemed to provide a principled way of identifying individuals whose problems lie *outside* the language production system, and distinctly performing groups of those whose production systems are impaired (though note that these individuals may also have have problems outside the system).

### Re-analysis of Crystal Data

The opportunity then arose to take advantage of data collected in the University Assessment Clinic at Reading, and analysed retrospectively by David Crystal as part of an MRC project (Crystal, 1986). This sample was thought to provide a stringent test for the framework of the earlier study. First, the new sample was more heterogeneous than that of our original study, in that no prior selection criteria are applied to children attending our Assessment Clinic, other than that they are considered language-impaired by a clinician. Also, since the clinic functions as a secondary referrral, the children who attend often have problems regarded as somewhat intractable. In addition, while for both studies the primary data were spontaneous speech, the protocols employed in collecting the data were different. Twenty-four of the children in Crystal's sample fell within the age-range of the earlier study (Fletcher, 1991), and the linguistic profiles and transcripts prepared by Crystal allowed the extraction of similar categories which could also be related to the language production model. Table 12.2 shows descriptive statistics for the variables involved.

Apart from age (note that subjects in the study ranged from 5;1 to 10;7) the variables require some annotation. COMPLEX and NOVPEXP measure stucture-building abilities; ERR is a measure of structure deployment difficulties, and FLUENCY is a measure of pause.

### Complex

This is the proportion of complex sentences appearing in the data for each subject. It is a general measure over three rather different types of clause linkage in English: more than one simple clause linked by a coordinator or subordinator indicating a particular semantic relationship; complex verb complementation; relative clauses.

**Table 12.2** Descriptive statistics and inter-correlations for variables AGE, COMPLEX, NPVPEXP, ERR and FLUENCY. Crystal, 1986 data

(a) Descriptive statistics

|         | Mean  | STDEV | Min   | Max  |
|---------|-------|-------|-------|------|
| Age     | 86.46 | 17.97 | 61    | 127  |
| Complex | 0.09  | 0.07  | 0.00. | 0.24 |
| Npvpexp | 1.02  | 0.33  | 0.27  | 1.85 |
| Err     | 0.53  | 0.52  | 0.07  | 2.71 |
| Fluency | 0.92  | 0.53  | 0.21  | 2.16 |

(b) Inter-correlations

|         | Age   | Compl | NPVP  | Err  |
|---------|-------|-------|-------|------|
| Complex | 0.37  |       |       |      |
| Npvpexp | −0.02 | 0.00  |       |      |
| Err     | −0.03 | −0.42 | −0.63 |      |
| Fluency | 0.08  | 0.02  | 0.47  | 0.28 |

*Npvpexp*

In any simple clause, a speaker has the choice of using phrasal or non-phrasal realisations for subject, object and complement, and also for verb and adverbial. This measure is the proportion of phrasal realisations per simple clause, and it is intended as an index of the amount of phrase structure the child is able to recruit, on-line, in constructing a sentence.

*Err*

This is a composite measure of syntactic and morphological errors appearing in the data, as represented in Stage VI of the LARSP chart (Crystal, Fletcher and Garman, 1990). The range of errors – incorrect verb argument structure, lexical selection problems, inappropriate systemic choice, omission of auxiliaries, determiners and inflections – are similar to those found in the earlier group analysed. Although not represented in Table 12.2, we did log separately errors that involved the omission of unstressed elements (auxiliary, copula, inflections), which we would want to attribute to the phonological encoding level of the model, and errors such as clause element omission, and inappropriate systemic choice, which we would want to locate in the grammatical encoder.

*Fluency*

This measure provides the proportion of pauses found within sentences.

It is clearly a general measure of fluency which may have more than one source in the speaker's beahaviour. We are assuming that at least one of the sources is lexical selection problems.

**Results and Discussion**

The correlations between age and the linguistic variables involved indicate no significant relationships here. Low correlations between the fluency variable and Complex and Error indicate that pause/search behaviour is independent of these also. There are, however, three significant correlations that need to be considered. Fluency and Npvpexp are negatively correlated, suggesting that there is a link between pause/search behaviour and structure-building. And Error is negatively correlated with both Complex and Npvpexp. So a subject who is more successful at structure building, measured in terms of frequency of successful utilisation of available syntactic patterns, is somewhat less likely to make mistakes in producing a sentence. Though the correlations are not very high, the measures that we are using to profile subjects, and to search for patterns of deficit, do not appear to be as independent of one another as those in the earlier study.

What happens when we look at how subjects are distributed across the dimensions of description that we have selected? The picture is unfortunately not as clear as it was in the earlier study, but nevertheless some general trends emerge which we can compare with the earlier results and also with Miller's proposed categories. If we use the same procedure as in the earlier study and identify, on each dimension, individuals at the extreme of the distribution, we can look for patterns. If we look at the dimensions separately, we find that about one-quarter of the subjects have a fluency problem, and about the same number are very prone to make errors in producing sentences. When we look for commonalities across subjects, the following tendencies emerge, accounting for about half the individuals involved.

1. There is a group of children who are relatively fluent, error-free and who have adequate structure building. The basis for this group's language impairment, like Group 1 in our earlier study, should be sought elsewhere than in the language production process. Again, we should consider Miller's discourse and semantic/referencing categories.

2. The second group is dysfluent, but has adequate structure building and is relatively error free. This may link in with Miller's Group 3, Rate and Fluency problems.

3. The third group is also dysfluent, and in addition has structure building problems with both Complex and Npvpexp, and is very prone to error on-line. It is possible that there is a subdivision here based on error types, with one subgroup having more problems with grammatical encoding, and another subgroup presenting with phonological encoding difficulties. Such subgroups would then correspond to our earlier Groups 2 and 3 in Table 12.1.

4. The third group is relatively fluent, and relatively free from error. They show structure-building problems, though in either Complex or Npvpexp, not both, which may mean that there are subgroups represented here also. This group does not correspond to any of the groups in Table 12.1.

In trying to summarise what we can make of all this I want to return once more to the first AFASIC symposium, this time to Michael Rutter's contribution. In his 'thoughts on causes and correlates', he was particularly concerned about heterogeneity in the population we are interested in, both in terms of aetiology and diagnostic classification. Clearly I cannot say anything about aetiology on the basis of these data. It does speak however to the issue of variability in the expression of whatever condition or conditions lie behind specific language impairment. Variability is not surprising. We would expect different adaptations to language disability, depending on such factors as age, intelligence, length and type of therapeutic intervention and so on. But because of the constraints of a finite linguistic system, expressed through a production apparatus with a specific structure, we would not expect the variability to be without limit –essentially for each subject to have a unique profile. Assuming also that language impairment is not reducible to impairment of some other cognitive system, it should be possible to identify children who evince similar behaviours in terms of their *language* behaviour exclusively. In attempting to do this, it is preferable to use a hypothesis-testing approach to classification. Our approach has been to adopt a process-oriented perspective on the characterisation of the expressive language of SLI children, and to link categories of description available from spontaneous speech data to the theroetical framework of a production model. The validation of a typology arising out of this theoretical framework will depend in part on its success at classifying subjects (internal validation), and in part on its external validation – its 'predictive, descriptive and clinical validity' (Wilson and Risucci, 1986). One of the advantages of a typology would be to provide a principled procedure for identifying children with different types of problems so that remediation could be targeted more effcetively. Another advantage would be for the exploration of links with potential aetiological factors.

This approach to variability, as so far developed, would seem to have a degree of internal validation, in terms of the proportion of children accounted for. It also in some measure reaches out to the clinical categories which have been suggested in the field. There is still, however, some way to go. In particular, the procedure we have outlined and which has been partially successful in profiling sub-groups needs to be subjected to an appropriate multivariate analysis, in which we would hope to account for more of the variance than we appear to be able to at present. It will be necessary, once we have done this for the language production process, to relate our findings to the children's comprehension ability. However it is our contention that the results so far support our view that considering the child's speech as the product of a complex of subsytems operating in real time offers the prospect of multidimensional profiling for the schoolage language-impaired child which is considerably more informative than the standard grammatical view.

## References

ARAM, D. and NATION, J. (1975). Patterns of language behaviour in children with developmental disorders. *Journal of Speech and Hearing Research*, 18, 229–241.

BISHOP, D. (1989). Autism, Asperger's syndrome and semantic–pragmatic disorder: where are the boundaries? *British Jounal of Disorders of Communication*, 24, 229–241.

CHIAT, S. and HIRSON, A. (1987). From conceptual intention to utterance: a study of impaired language output in a child with developmental dysphasia. *British Jounal of Disorders of Communication*, 22, 37–64.

CRAIN, S., MCKEE, C. and EMILIANI, M. (1990).Visiting relatives in Italy. In: Frazier, L. and de Villiers, J (Eds), *Language Processing and Language Acquisition*, pp. 335–356. Kluwer Academic Publishers.

CRYSTAL, D. (1986). The diagnosis of language disorders in children. Final Report on MRC grant no. G8306096NA.

CRYSTAL, D., FLETCHER, P. and GARMAN, M. (1990). *The Grammatical Analysis of Language Disability: A Procedure for Assessment and Remediation*, 2nd edn. London: Whurr Publishers.

CURTISS, S. and TALLAL, P. (1991). On the nature of the impairment in language-impaired children. In: Millar, J. (Ed), *Research in Child Language Disorders: A Decade of Progress*, pp. 189–210. Austin, TX: Pro-Ed.

FLETCHER, P. (1991). Evidence from syntax for language impairment. In: Miller, J. (Ed.), *Research in Child Language Disorders: A Decade of Progress*, pp. 169–188. Austin, TX: Pro-Ed.

LEVELT, W. (1989). *Speaking: From Intention to Articulation*. Cambridge, MA.: MIT Press.

LIEBERMAN, P. (1991). *Uniquely Human: The Evolution of Speech, Thought and Selfless Behaviour*. Cambridge, MA: Harvard University Press.

MARTIN, J.A.M., FLETCHER, P., GRUNWELL, P. and HALL, D. (1987). *Proceedings of the First International Symposium on Specific Speech and Language Disorders in Children*. London: AFASIC (Association for all Speech Impaired Children).

MILLER, J. (1987). A grammatical characterisation of language disorder. In: Martin, J.A.M., Fletcher, P., Grunwell,P. and Hall, D. (Eds), *Proceedings of the First International Symposium on Specific Speech and Language Disorders in Children*. London: AFASIC.

RAPIN, I. (1982). *Children with Brain Dysfunction*. New York: Raven Press.

RAPIN, I. and ALLEN, D. (1982). Developmental language disorders: nosologic considerations. In: Kirk, V. (Ed.), *Neuropsychology of Language, Reading and Spelling*. New York: Academic Press.

WILSON, B. and RISUCCI, D. (1986). A model for clinical-quantitative classification. Generation I: application to language-disordered pre-school children. *Brain and Language*, 27, 281–309.

WOLFUS, B., MOSCOVITCH, M. and KINSBOURNE, M. (1980). Subgroups of developmental language impairment. *Brain and Language*, 10, 152–171.

WREN, C. (1980). Identifying patterns of language disorder. In: *Proceedings of the First Wisconsin Symposium on Research in Child Language Disorders*. Madison: University of Wisconsin–Madison.

# Part IV

# Outcomes, Intervention and the Curriculum

# Chapter 13
# A longitudinal study of language-impaired children from a residential school

**CORINNE HAYNES**

This paper is concerned with 156 pupils at one of the very few special schools in the UK and probably within the world, for children with severe and specific speech and language impairment.

In 1974, language units were just beginning to open in some numbers in this country, in the expectation that 2–3 years of special education and speech therapy would enable language-impaired children to return to mainstream education. At this time, Invalid Children's Aid Nationwide (I CAN), the voluntary body which had since 1959 administered the John Horniman School for SLI pupils aged between 5 and 9 had come to a different decision. As a result of a follow-up study of John Horniman pupils (Griffiths, 1969), which found that pupils who had apparently overcome their oral language problems were showing continuing educational and social problems after return to mainstream schools, I CAN decided to extend their own provision and opened Dawn House school in Nottinghamshire to cater for 54 day and residential pupils up to 13 years of age. As therapists and teachers at Dawn House worked closely with these children, the persistent and broad nature of their problems became increasingly clear, and in 1987 a secondary department was opened, allowing some pupils to remain at Dawn House until they reached school-leaving age at 16. It is with the long-term and pervasive nature of the difficulties of the SLI child that this chapter is concerned.

Detailed records are kept at Dawn House of each child's developmental, social, medical, educational and language history. Both the first head-teacher of the school, Sandhya Naidoo, an educational psychologist, and myself, a speech and language therapist, felt that these records should be used rather than stored in ever increasing numbers of filing cabinets. In the hope of gaining some useful insights into the nature of the problems of these special children, in 1987 we set up a computer database with around 1000 variables entered for each subject.

The school has entry criteria which exclude children below a set level of non-verbal intelligence, hearing level and emotional–behavioural status with the aim of achieving a relatively homogeneous population, but inevitably the demarcation lines get a little blurred and special exceptions are made in case of need. For our research study we tried to keep our group reasonably 'pure' and excluded children on the borderline of our criteria. This left us with a group of 156 children who had entered the school between 1974 and 1987 (Table 13.1).

Table 13.1 Children in the study by age at entry and gender

|  | Age (years) | | | | |
|---|---|---|---|---|---|
|  | 5;0–6;11 | 7;0–8;11 | 9;0–10;11 | 11;0–12;11 | Total |
| Boys | 42 | 60 | 27 | 0 | 129 |
| Girls | 9 | 8 | 8 | 2 | 27 |
| Total | 51 | 68 | 35 | 2 | 156 |

Mean age at entry 7;10.

## Description of Children

Children who come into school have a wide range of language and speech impairments at the perceptual, conceptual, semantic, syntactic, phonological and articulatory levels that prevent the development of normal communication and interfere with their ability to benefit from mainstream education. They are all willing to communicate, have normal non-verbal intelligence and hearing within normal limits. If these conditions are met they are candidates for entry. Age range at entry was from 5;2 years to 12;10, mean 7;10, and at leaving from 6;10 years to 13;10, mean 11;9. The ratio of boys to girls was 4.8:1.

### Language Abilities at Entry

On entry to school children's oral language abilities are assessed by the speech therapists. In the 16 years since Dawn House opened the characterisation of normal and abnormal language has undergone several revisions, and not only the 'how' but also the 'what' of assessments has changed considerably. In order to achieve some consistency in describing the children's disabilities we have had to limit our examination of results to tests which were current in 1974 and still in use today, and operate within the 1970s polarised theoretical framework of comprehension and expression, reporting separately on speech and written language abilities. The tests that meet these conditions are presented in Table 13.2.

**Table 13.2** Language assessments recorded at entry

| | |
|---|---|
| *Comprehension* | |
| Vocabulary | English Picture Vocabulary Test |
| | British Picture Vocabulary Scale |
| Grammar | Test for Reception of Grammar |
| General | Reynell Developmental Language Scale |
| | |
| *Production* | |
| Vocabulary | Renfrew Word-Finding Scale |
| Structure | LARSP |
| Morphology | Grammatic Closure (ITPA) |
| Content | Renfrew Bus Story |
| | |
| *Speech* | |
| Maturity | Edinburgh Articulation Raw Score |
| Deviance | Edinburgh Articulation Atypical Score |
| | |
| *Written Language* | |
| Reading Age | Southgate Group Reading Tests |

All of these assessments measure different language skills, and in the research report (Haynes and Naidoo, 1991), we examine the relationship of each language ability with a range of possible antecedent factors, such as family history of language impairment and birth history, and also with correlates such as auditory memory, intelligence and laterality. However, a recurring problem with retrogressive research, for which data collection has not been preplanned, is that not all of the children have done all of the tests, and datasets are therefore incomplete. To get round this problem where it was essential to have a comparable measure for each child, we calculated some composite scores for comprehension, expression and speech based on scores of the available tests. Generally we categorised scores of less than one standard deviation below the norm as normal or minor impairment, from one to two as moderate, and below two as severe, within each of the language areas of comprehension, expression and speech. The terms 'minor' and 'moderate' are of course relative, since all children coming to Dawn House have major language problems. There were too many non-readers to produce a similar banding for written language.

## Subgroups

In spite of our efforts to cut off the most extreme outliers of our sample, our group of children was far from homogeneous, and it seemed likely that much potential interest in analysis could be lost by treating them as a single entity. We were also – like most researchers before us and doubtless many more still to come – keen to isolate some groups which had some sort of clinical validity. As practitioners at the sharp end we wanted group divisions that would be pertinent when we had to organise classes or set therapy goals. We felt that we had one advantage over more academic researchers in that, as teacher–psychologist and speech–language therapist, we had personally assessed every child coming into school and had been involved in working with most of them. This put us in a good position to combine clinical insight with objective test results in grouping children into disability subgroups, and this is what we did, beginning with clinically intuitive grouping, then examining the test profiles of children so grouped, and finally grading all children according to the most coherent objective group profiles. This finally produced the nine subgroups shown in Table 13.3.

The slightly odd names need glossing. They are simply descriptive, and although they may correspond to previously described taxonomies– our Classic group for example resembles Rapin and Allen's (1983) Phonologic–Syntactic syndrome – they do not do so on the basis of any agreed criteria. Since they encapsulate a profile of impairment based upon the relationship of three broad linguistic skills, they can be represented as in Figure 13.1.

A child in the Speech group has relatively minor language, as opposed to speech, difficulties. For the Speech plus child, speech is still the worst affected communication skill, but his expressive and also possibly his

**Table 13.3** Subgroups of language impairment

|  | *n* | Comprehension | Expression | Speech |
| --- | --- | --- | --- | --- |
| Speech | 19 | Minor | Minor | Severe |
| Speech plus | 23 | Minor/moderate | Moderate | Severe |
| Classic | 46 | Minor/moderate | Severe | Moderate/severe |
| Semantic | 30 | Moderate/severe | Minor/moderate/severe | Minor/moderate |
| Residual | 10 | Minor/moderate | Minor/moderate | Minor/moderate |
| Moderate | 13 | Minor/moderate | Minor/moderate | Minor/moderate |
| No language | 6 | Severe | Severe | Severe |
| Young unclassified | 6 | Severe | Severe | Severe |
| Severe | 3 | Severe | Severe | Severe |

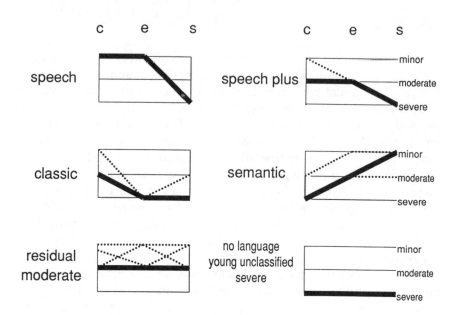

**Figure 13.1** Profiles of language subgroups

comprehensive skills are worse than those of the Speech child. The Classic child has the profile most often thought of in connection with SLI, with expressive language most severely affected, and this is our largest group. The defining feature of the Semantic group is that comprehension is always at the lowest point of the profile. The next two groups have identical profiles and we have separated ten of them into a Residual rather than a Moderate group because they had come to us from other language schools and units, and we felt that their profiles at entry might have been raised because of this; they could actually be improved members of some other category. The last three groups all have the same profile, and to some extent this reflects the insensitivity of most assessments for the most handicapped children. All these children performed at rock bottom in all areas and we have separated them for clinical reasons. The No language group entered school with no means of communication and so could not be profiled using standard instruments. The Young unclassified are just that, children of 5 or 6 years with some limited communication, whose very delayed start did not necessarily predict future profiles. Finally the Severe group comprises children with the same profile of minimal ability but aged 7 or above, which we took to be an indicator of serious and persisting handicap.

National and local educational policies change, and the type of SLI child for whom LEAs make application to Dawn House has changed during its 16 years of existence. Current pupils are often more broadly handicapped and require longer in special education than our original intake. Over the 13 years of the study the mean length of stay was 3 years 9 months, and ranged from 11 months to 6 years 11 months.

## Intervention

There are no comparative treatment groups. Over a period of 13 years approaches have obviously been changing and refining. Also the balance of disabilities within the school population is not constant so that sometimes we have had a large enough group of Semantic children to form a special class and sometimes we have not. What has remained constant is the general philosophy and approach which I will briefly summarise.

Children are taught in small classes of 6–10. Speech–language therapists work with caseloads of 10 or 11 children, usually with particular class groups. Juniors board in family units of eight children with a houseparent; seniors of 12 years and older board in a larger house with facilities for teenage pursuits. All staff involved with a child are concerned with social and language development and meet to discuss, plan and evaluate this. Children can use any means to communicate as language develops. A manual sign system, Paget–Gorman, is learned by all staff and used as a language teaching aid. Children make use of this system according to need and level of development. They should always speak – or at least vocalise – when they sign. We believe strongly that an integrated approach is most effective where learning is so laborious. Teachers, therapists, therapy aides and classroom assistants work closely together and their professional roles become blurred. For direct language work we aim to reduce any unnecessary load on processing and memory, to provide sufficient small steps, and to make the work relevant and enjoyable, thus enabling the child to become an active language learner. Daily sessions of oral language work in small groups of two to four concentrate on specific aspects of language skill according to current needs. Reading and writing activities are kept to the level of each child's oral language development. Since our principal aim is meaningful and confident communication, we encourage the use of strategies to circumvent persistent language problems such as word-finding difficulties, and increasingly work to develop communicative social skills and foster self-esteem.

## Outcomes

Of the 156 children in the sample, 118 had left Dawn House or moved into the senior school when the study began. In addition to a battery of language and scholastic tests which space does not allow me to describe here, three broad measures were used to assess outcomes of the 118 leavers. These are language, speech and reading, each of which was rated from 1 to 3, as good, fair and poor.

*Language Outcome*

Children attend Dawn House because their language difficulties are too severe for them to achieve their potential in mainstream school. If they improve sufficiently to return to mainstream, they are deemed to have a good language outcome; 52% of leavers were in this category. Children who still required education in language school after reaching our (previous) leaving age of 13 were deemed to have a poor language outcome and 40% of leavers were in this category. A further 8% fell between these two positions, no longer requiring education oriented to language disability but not yet able to benefit from mainstream. These children, rated fair for language outcome, went to other special schools offering some additional support (see Table 13.4).

*Speech Outcome*

The speech component of outcome relates both to intelligibility and to the completeness of the phonological system. Thus children with some minor immaturities of the r/w type, or having some difficulty with polysyllables could obtain a good rating, but children with atypical sound substitutions which are noticeably odd, could not. Final speech outcomes are detailed in Table 13.5.

**Table 13.4** Language outcome

|       | No. | Percentage | Criteria |
|-------|-----|------------|----------|
| Good  | 62  | 52         | Can return to mainstream |
| Fair  | 9   | 8          | Additional support in other special schools |
| Poor  | 47  | 40         | Still require language school |
| Total | 118 | 100        | |

**Table 13.5** Speech outcome

|       | No. | Percentage | Criteria (Edinburgh Articulation Test) | |
|-------|-----|------------|-----------|----------|
|       |     |            | Raw score | Atypical |
| Good  | 72  | 61         | 50 +      | <2       |
| Fair  | 10  | 8          | 33–49     | <2       |
| Poor  | 36  | 31         | <33       | 2+       |
| Total | 118 | 100        |           |          |

*Reading Outcome*

Most of our leavers still need remedial reading support, but some achieve serviceable levels of reading and others, at still earlier stages of reading, are functioning at levels close to average for age. Many others have by any criterion a serious reading problem. The most meaningful way to measure outcome in reading seemed to be a combination of reading age with the difference between reading and chronological age. The criteria for good, fair and poor outcomes, which are of course relative to this sample and not a normal population, are shown in Table 13.6.

*Overall Outcome Grade*

Finally, and mainly for the purposes of statistical analysis, we combined all these outcome components into a single final outcome grade as follows:

1. Good
   Language and speech outcomes good. Reading good or fair.
2. Fair
   One component good. Language no worse than fair. No more than one component poor.
3. Poor
   Two components rated poor, or one poor and two fair.

Of 118 leavers, using these criteria 32% had a good outcome, 35% had a fair outcome and 33% had a poor outcome.

**Table 13.6** Reading outcome

|        | No. | Percentage | Criteria |
|--------|-----|------------|----------|
| Good   | 22  | 19         | RA 10;0+ or CA-RA < 1 |
| Fair   | 52  | 44         | Children aged 10 years or under, RA 7;6+ CA-RA 12–30 months |
|        |     |            | Children over 10 years RA 7;6+ CA-RA 12–48 months |
| Poor   | 44  | 37         | Children aged 10 years or under RA <7;6 CA–RA >30 months |
|        |     |            | Children over 10 years RA <7;6, CA-RA >48 months |
| Total  | 118 | 100        |          |

RA, reading age; CA-RA, chronological age-reading age

One goal of this research was to judge whether prediction of outcome was possible from the information gathered and assessments made at entry. Using the developmental history information and results of tests at entry which are fully described in the research report (Haynes and Naidoo 1991), we were able to predict outcome accurately according to the three categories I have described here, in 70% of cases.

**Subgroups and Outcome**

We were interested in looking at the outcome of our various subgroups. If outcome proved to relate to subgroup membership, not only might we be able to improve prognosis at entry, but this would also to some extent validate the subgroups that we had demarcated.

The final outcome grade (which combines the language, speech and reading outcome components) is shown in Figure 13.2 for each subgroup, arranged in order of best to worst outcome.

The best outcome was in the Residual group. Of nine leavers in this group eight had a good and one a fair outcome. We had originally argued that this group of children might represent a more handicapped population than the Moderate group whose entry profile they shared, and that some years of previous special language help could have raised their profile. If this were the case, one would have expected a final outcome similar to the large groups such as the Classic or Semantic. In practice they outperformed both of these groups; nor can their good outcome necessarily be attributed to additional years of special help, since their stay at Dawn House was shorter than average, making the overall period of special education similar to other groups. We re-examined our data

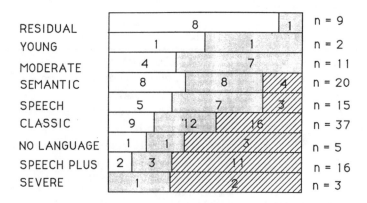

**Figure 13.2** Outcome grades proportionally by subgroup. □ Good; ▨ fair; ▨ poor.

and concluded that these were probably less handicapped children than those normally entering Dawn House, and that they had come from establishments with different entry criteria.

I have included the Young unclassified only for the sake of completeness. They were not in any real diagnostic category and there are only two leavers, so there is no useful information to trawl from this result.

The Moderate handicap group had a reasonably good outcome as expected.

Some of our most puzzling children are in the Semantic group, for whom comprehension is the worst affected language area. Our rather gross definition is inadequate to characterise this group of children with sometimes quite subtle difficulties, who tend to have peaks and troughs of ability. On the whole the outcome is reasonably good, with 80% having a good or fair outcome. Looking at the individual components, language outcome is about half good and half poor, speech (which is not a major problem in this group) is generally good, and reading generally poor.

The Speech group were expected to have a good outcome. Bishop and Edmundson (1987a) argued that a narrow rather than a broad spectrum of language disability had a better prognosis, and several previous longitudinal studies have found better outcome in articulation-impaired than in language-impaired groups (Hall and Tomblin 1978; King, Jones and Lasky, 1982). Our Speech group did moderately well. Almost all returned to mainstream education, but around half had some persisting speech problems and over half had a continuing reading difficulty.

We anticipated that the Classic children would have long-lasting and pervasive difficulties. This is the most archetypal subgroup of SLI described in the literature. Over 40% had a poor outcome, almost half needing to continue in special language school after age 13. Speech outcome was satisfactory, 65% having a good outcome, while severe reading difficulties persisted in nearly half of the leavers.

The No language and Severe groups are very small but seem to indicate, as expected, continuing major difficulties.

A surprising result is the outcome of the Speech plus subgroup. These children had a not dissimilar profile to the Speech group at entry. Both groups had severe speech problems but the Speech plus had additional moderate language problems where the Speech group had only minor language impairment. We expected them to do only a little less well than the Speech children, but in fact they had much poorer outcomes. There were some indications from the analysis, which I have not space to explore further here, that this particular group of children could have distinct speech and language handicaps with separate aetiologies. They proved to be among our most handicapped children.

## Follow-up at 18+

At the time of the study pupils left Dawn House at the age of 13 years or before. Normally, 1–2 years after leaving, we asked for reports from home and school. After that, with the exception of those few parents, and even fewer pupils, who kept in touch, we had no knowledge of how they were progressing. It seemed important to find out. An effort was made to contact the 43 young people in the study who had reached the age of 18. Contact was established with 34 of them, and a telephone questionnaire was put to either the young person, or if they so chose, to one of their parents.

We were interested generally in how they were getting on in life compared with other young people of the same age, and specifically in how they had fared educationally since leaving Dawn House, in their work and career opportunities, and in their social life. We also asked for their own opinion of their language abilities both currently and while at school. We questioned 26 young men and 8 young women or their parents. Their age ranged from 18;5 to 22;10 at the time of the follow-up.

### Education After Dawn House

All these young people had left Dawn House before the senior department opened. Table 13.7 shows the type of education which followed next and public examination results. About 60% had gone on to sit public examinations, and these were largely the children who had been able to return to mainstream schools.

Although previous studies have indicated that continuing educational problems are more often found in language-impaired than articulation-impaired individuals (Hall and Tomblin, 1978), if we look at these educational attainments in terms of our subgroups we see a range of attainment across groups, with the Speech and the Moderate groups possibly having the most success (Table 13.8). All the individuals who went on to

**Table 13.7** Education and examinations of follow-up pupils

|            | No. | GCE-A   | GCE-O   | CSE      | None |
|------------|-----|---------|---------|----------|------|
| Mainstream | 22  | 3(2–4)* | 5(1–12) | 15(1–7)  | 7    |
| Language   | 7   |         |         | 4(1-3)   | 3    |
| MLD        | 4   |         |         | 1(1)     | 3    |
| Private    | 1   |         |         | 1(4)     | –    |
| Total      | 34  | 3       | 5       | 21       | 13   |

GCE-O, GCE-A, General Certificate of Education, Ordinary and Advanced Level; CSE, Certificate of Secondary Education; MLD, Moderate Learning Difficulty; *Figures in brackets indicate number of papers taken.

**Table 13.8** Exam results by subgroup

|  | No. | Total GCE * | | Mean CSE |
| --- | --- | --- | --- | --- |
|  |  | O-level | A-level |  |
| Speech | 4 | 6 | 4 | 3.00 |
| Speech plus | 3 |  |  | 0.60 |
| Classic | 14 | 1 |  | 2.10 |
| Semantic | 4 | 12 | 2 | 0.25 |
| Residual | 3 | 6 | 3 | 1.00 |
| Moderate | 3 | 3 |  | 5.30 |
| No language | 3 |  |  | 1.30 |
| Total | 34 | 28 | 9 | 2.10 |

* GCE O and A levels were obtained by five individual children.

attain the more academic GCE results were pupils who attended in the 1970s. It is doubtful whether local authorities would sponsor these pupils in special education today, and according to their parents, it is doubtful whether without the special educational start the pupils would have achieved their eventual success.

*Tertiary Education*

About one-third of the group had no tertiary education, the remainder had further education which varied from university or polytechnic for the three pupils with A -level attainments, to some College day-release as part of a Youth Training Scheme. Many of the further education courses available for language-impaired individuals are not appropriate, being designed for slow learners. Some of our youngsters had become very disillusioned, having looked forward expectantly to college life, to find that they were repeating work already done at school, but at a slower pace. There is currently a gap in provision for SLI youngsters aged 16–20, and I understand that AFASIC is investigating the possibility of improving this.

*Work*

Twenty-five youngsters were employed at the time of the questionnaire and four were students. Of the five unemployed, two seemed to be genuinely between jobs, one not accepting contract work that was too far from home and one being laid off while work was short. The other three had only done temporary or no jobs, and were probably long-term unemployed. The range of work was varied (see Table 13.9) but with an emphasis on manual or partly skilled work. Those who had participated in government training schemes such as YTS, had statistically a slightly

**Table 13.9** Employment by subgroup

Speech
  Engineering storekeeper
  Degree student–electronic engineering
  Clerical work
  Market trader (self-employed)

Speech plus
  Building labourer
  Soap packer
  Unemployed

Classic
  Nurseryman                          Student catering course
  Bar work                            Greengrocery assistant
  Gardener                            Garden ornament painter
  P/T catering assitant (3)           Livestock farmer (self-employed)
  Temporary catering assistant        Brusher-off in clothing factory
  Kitchen porter                      Unemployed

Semantic
  Classroom assistant
  Degree student  – economics
  Building labourer
  Unemployed

Residual
  Vehicle recovery driver
  Degree student – physics
  Unemployed

Moderate
  Electrician
  Crane driver
  Cabinet maker

No language
  Fibreglass moulder
  Kitchen assistant
  Unemployed

better chance of being in employment. As with the further educational courses, the training programmes offered to SLI youngsters were frequently at a low level; four were in skilled occupations, nine in partly skilled and eight in unskilled work. One young man whose non-verbal IQ at Dawn House had been about 130 had been excited when placed with a company producing holographs. Over the telephone to me, he explained very coherently the way holographs were made. He left the firm when he discovered that his training was confined to sweeping the floor, wiping down the equipment and making tea, and is now disillusioned and unemployed.

When we originally looked at the social class mix of the families of our 156 subjects, we found that it resembled that of the general population but with an increase of manual as opposed to non-manual workers in Social Group III. This would be consonant with the familial pattern of language difficulties which we also report. It seemed possible that the high level of manual work obtained by our follow-up subjects was similar to their families' work pattern. Table 13.10 shows that this is not so. There is a downward movement in socioeconomic status, some of which I suggest is due not to the actual abilities of these young people, but to the expectations held by others of the capabilities of those whose language sounds a little unusual.

### Social Life and Residual Problems

Some of our questionnaires were answered by our ex-pupils and some by their parents. When we had the opportunity we spoke to both and it was interesting that in these two areas – social life and residual difficulties – we had different replies, depending on the respondent.

Family life was still central to most of these young people. Twenty-nine lived at home and the remainder were in student accommodation

Table 13.10 Socioeconomic status of follow-up group compared with their families

|                    | Family | Subject |
|--------------------|--------|---------|
| Top professional   | 4      | 0       |
| Managerial         | 3      | 1       |
| Skilled non-manual | 3      | 2       |
| Skilled manual     | 17     | 5       |
| Partly skilled     | 6      | 9       |
| Unskilled          | 1      | 8       |
| Unemployed         | 0      | 5       |
| (Students)         | –      | 4       |
| Total              | 34     | 34      |

or living with relatives or family friends. Many relied quite considerably on the social groups of which their families were part. Twenty youngsters went out regularly with friends of their own age, but 14 did so only rarely, or had only older or younger companions. Only two out of 17 youngsters questioned admitted to difficulties socially; but of 21 parents asked the same question regarding the social skills of their offspring, 13 reported problems. We feel that both of these viewpoints could be over-reporting. Very few teenagers may feel able to say openly that socially they are not successful. Similarly we feel that parents of any handicapped child are all too aware of that child's difficulties, and may give some emotional charge to a social situation – loneliness or relative isolation – that the parent of a young person without special problems would con-sider less abnormal. One further point to bear in mind here is age. This is a population of young people who may still be neurodevelopmentally lagging behind (Bishop and Edmundson, 1987b). Certainly they are not the equals of their peers when social and communicative skills are mea-sured. It is probably more realistic to compare their social achievements with those of adolescents some 2–3 years younger, than with their chronological peers.

The final statistic concerns residual difficulties. At the beginning of this paper I cited the view, prevalent in the 1970s, that some intensive special help during the formative years would relocate SLI children in the mainstream of their peer group. Our report of the further education, career and social prospects of children with severe and specific lan-guage impairment gives the lie to that belief. Only three of the 34 young people or their parents considered that there were no residual difficul-ties of any sort with either spoken or written language. The specific diffi-culties reported are shown by subgroup in Table 13.11. Most difficulties are reported with speaking and spelling. Many of them may be relatively minor; quoted difficulties are the pronunciation of 'big words', using the

**Table 13.11** Residual problems by subgroup

|               | Comprehension | Expression | Speech | Reading | Writing | Spelling |
|---------------|:---:|:---:|:---:|:---:|:---:|:---:|
| Speech (*n*=4)   | 0  | 2  | 4  | 0  | 1  | 3  |
| Speech (*n*=3)   | 2  | 2  | 1  | 0  | 1  | 3  |
| Classic (*n*=14) | 6  | 9  | 9  | 8  | 9  | 8  |
| Semantic (*n*=4) | 2  | 1  | 3  | 1  | 1  | 2  |
| Residual (*n*=3) | 2  | 2  | 2  | 1  | 2  | 2  |
| Moderate (*n*=3) | 1  | 1  | 2  | 0  | 1  | 2  |
| No lang. (*n*=3) | 3  | 2  | 3  | 3  | 2  | 1  |
| TOTAL (*n*=34)   | 16 | 19 | 24 | 13 | 17 | 21 |

telephone, and following films, problems that many people might experience who have never had a language impairment. Nevertheless, if these are considered to be noteworthy problems by the young people, they may well affect their confidence and ability to relax socially.

The impression grew upon us in conducting the follow up, that a successful outcome in terms of a full and satisfactory life, did not require faultless communication skills, but did depend upon a measure of self-confidence and social *savoir faire*. Our data on social and emotional strengths of pupils are not very objective, being drawn from the biannual reports of school and house staff while the child attended Dawn House, but it is based on several years of informed observation. We compared the 14 subjects from our follow-up group who seemed to have most friends and a range of sociable pursuits with the 13 who reported social difficulties on a range of early variables including extent and type of language disability, whether they had been boarders or day pupils, and the (school) behaviour clusters of solitariness, peer relationships, confidence, attitude to communication and coping with difficulties. The one variable that seemed best to separate the two groups was attitude to communication. Those subjects who had been ready and eager to communicate at school, regardless of the extent of their language handicap were more likely as young adults to be enjoying satisfactory social relationships.

## Summary

Pupils with severe language impairment were categorised by a combination of clinical observation and objective measures. Standard assessments were not adequate to describe the children with the greatest handicaps. The difference in outcome for groups whose entry profiles (based on tests alone) were similar underlines the advisability of using a combined clinical objective appraisal.

If given appropriate and intensive help, it is possible for some SLI children to make excellent progress and achieve great success, but for almost all some language difficulties persist and for many these problems will affect scholastic achievement, work prospects and social life.

As professionals involved with language handicapped people, we often make a plea for increased awareness and acceptance within the community for people suffering from language impairments. We clearly need to continue to make this plea, but equally important, and possibly easier to achieve, is the positive acceptance by language-impaired youngsters and their families of a difference – rather than a deficit – which need cause neither shame nor despair, and which should not diminish self-esteem.

I hope to see language-impaired young people leave our schools and units knowing that they deal with sounds, words and sentences a little differently from their neighbour, but feeling for all that not one whit less able to take a full and equal place in society.

## Appendix: Tests and Suppliers

British Picture Vocabulary Scale. (Dunn et al.,1982). Windsor: NFER-Nelson.

The Bus Story (Renfrew, C.,1969). Available from the author, North Place, Old Headington, Oxford

Edinburgh Articulation Test (Anthony et al.,1971). Edinburgh: Churchill Livingstone.

Illinois Test of Psycholinguistic Abilities (Kirk et al.,1968). Windsor: NFER-Nelson.

Language Assessment, Remediation and Screening Procedure (LARSP). In: Crystal, D., Fletcher, P. and Garman, M.(1976) The Grammatical Assessment of Language Disability. London: Edward Arnold

Reynell Developmental Language Scales – Revised (Reynell,1977). Windsor: NFER-Nelson.

Southgate Group Reading Tests (Southgate, 1976). Sevenoaks, Kent: Hodder & Stoughton.

Test for Reception of Grammar (TROG) (Bishop, D., 1983). Available from the author, Department of Psychology, University of Manchester.

Word Finding Vocabulary Scale (Renfrew, C., 1972). Available from the author, North Place, Old Headington, Oxford.

## References

BISHOP, D.V. M. and EDMUNDSON, A. (1987a). Language impaired 4-year-olds: distinguishing transient from persistent impairment. *Journal of Speech and Hearing Disorders,* 52(2),156–173.

BISHOP, D.V. M. and EDMUNDSON, A. (1987b). Specific language impairment as a maturational lag; evidence from longitudinal data on language and motor development. *Developmental Medicine and Child Neurology* , 29, 442–459

GRIFFITHS, C.P.S. (1969). A follow-up study of children with disorders of speech. *British Journal of Disorders of Communication,* 4, 46–56

HALL, P. K. and TOMBLIN, J. B. (1978). A follow-up study of children with articulation and language disorders. *Journal of Speech and Hearing Disorders,* 43, 227–241.

HAYNES, C.P.A and NAIDOO, S. (1991). Children with Specific Speech and Language Impairment. *Clinics in Developmental Medicine No. 119.* London: MacKeith Press.

KING, R.R., JONES, C. and LASKY, E. (1982). In retrospect: a fifteen year follow-up report of speech-language disordered children. *Language, Speech and Hearing Services in Schools,* 13(1), 24–32.

RAPIN, I. and ALLEN, D. (1983). Developmental language disorders: nosological considerations. In: Kirk, U. (Ed.), *Neuropsychology of Language, Reading and Spelling.* New York: Academic Press.

# Chapter 14
# Reading and writing skills in the National Curriculum

KATHARINE PERERA

## Introduction: The National Curriculum

Since 1990, England and Wales have, for the first time, had a legally enforceable National Curriculum in English. This is not a detailed syllabus but rather a framework for the knowledge, skills and understanding that pupils should have acquired by four key stages in their schooling, which correspond roughly to ages 7, 11, 14 and 16. Children with special educational needs may be exempted from specific requirements of the curriculum; for example, those with a severe phonological disorder will need the oral requirements of the curriculum to be modified. Nevertheless, it is the government's intention that, as much as possible of the English curriculum should be available to all pupils:

> We believe ... that competence in English is important, both in its own right and to enable pupiles to gain access to and benefit from the other subects of the National Curriculum. Pupils with special educational needs ... should have the opportunity to experience as far as possible the full range of the English curriculum. For example, pupils with reading problems ... should not be deprived of literature, but should have the opportunity of experiencing it through listening to others reading aloud ... as well as through reading suitably simplified versions.
>
> (DES, 1989; Cox, 1991*)

*The National Curriculum in English is closely based on the Report of the English Working Group, which appeared in 1989 and which – because the Group was chaired by Professor Brian Cox – was popularly known as the Cox Report. This Report is no longer available (and was never available outside Great Britain), but it has been incorporated within a book by Brian Cox (1991). Therefore, when I quote from the Report, I shall give both the original source and the more accessible reference.

For the purposes of reporting pupils' performance to parents, the content of the English curriculum is divided into three Profile Components: Speaking and Listening, Reading, and Writing. Each Profile Component consists of one or more Attainment Targets (ATs). There is one for Speaking and Listening, one for Reading and three for Writing; these are the ATs for Reading and Writing:

*Profile Component Reading, Attainment Target 2:* 'The development of the ability to read, understand and respond to all types of writing, as well as the development of information-retrieval strategies for the purposes of study.' (DES, 1989; Cox, 1991)
*Profile Component Writing, Attainment Target 3:* 'A growing ability to construct and convey meaning in written language matching style to audience and purpose.' (DES, 1989; Cox, 1991)
*Profile Component Writing, Attainment Target 4:* Spelling (DES, 1989; Cox, 1991)
*Profile Component Writing, Attainment Target 5:* Handwriting (DES, 1989; Cox, 1991)

Within ATs 2 and 3, the knowledge, skills and understanding that are expected are divided into ten levels, with level 1 representing the attainment of the average 5-year-old after a term in school, level 4 being normal for an 11-year-old at the end of the primary school and levels 6/7 being typical of the average 16-year-old school leaver. At each level, the curriculum is expressed in terms of a number of 'statements of attainment'. For example, AT3 (Writing) has four statements of attainment at level 2:

Pupils should be able to:
(a) produce, independently, pieces of writing using complete sentences, some of them demarcated with capital letters and full stops or question marks;
(b) structure sequences of real or imagined events coherently in chronological accounts;
(c) write stories showing an understanding of the rudiments of story structure by establishing an opening, characters, and one or more events;
(d) produce simple, coherent non-chronological writing.

(DES, 1989; Cox, 1991)

Generally speaking, a pupil has to be able to meet every statement at a given level within a particular AT in order to be judged to have achieved that level on the AT. The individual statements of attainment represent strands within the curriculum; as such, they can be traced through the levels. For example, the 'non-chronological writing' strand that is introduced at level 2 continues like this at levels 3 and 4:

*Level 3* 'produce a range of types of non-chronological writing.' (DES, 1989; Cox, 1991)

*Level 4* 'organise non-chronological writing for different purposes in orderly ways.' (DES, 1989; Cox, 1991)

The statements of attainment set out what pupils are expected to achieve. The other crucial component of the curriculum is the programmes of study that are designed to support each AT. These set out what teachers need to do in order to ensure that pupils can fulfil the statements of attainment at the appropriate level. Both the programmes of study and the statements of attainment deal extensively with the skills of reading and writing. There are, for example, 42 separate statements of attainment that together constitute AT3 in writing and 50 for AT2 in reading. It would clearly not be feasible to deal with all 92 of these in this chapter. Therefore, I shall present just one general principle that applies to both the reading and the writing attainment targets; then I shall exemplify it from the statements of attainment and programmes of study; and finally I shall suggest some of the difficulties that might arise for those pupils who have language or literacy problems, and briefly outline some ways of meeting those difficulties.

## Varieties of Text Types

A theme that runs throughout the English curriculum is the need for pupils to have experience of a wide variety of kinds of written language. For example, in reading, 'it is necessary for children to have plenty of opportunities to read or hear read good examples of a range of different types of texts.' (DES, 1989; Cox, 1991). In addition to the familiar stories and poems, pupils need to be introduced to transactional uses of print: the Cox Report states that, 'schools have an obligation to help them to read everything from labels and slogans to the subject textbooks of the secondary school curriculum' (DES, 1989; Cox, 1991).

As far as writing is concerned, all primary teachers are used to teaching pupils to write diaries and stories as well as accounts of topic work that they have carried out in the classroom. But for some time it has been a matter of concern that some pupils are not being encouraged to produce a sufficiently wide range of kinds of writing. For example, a report in 1987 by the Assessment of Performance Unit concluded, 'The evidence gathered from successive surveys of pupils' attitudes to reading and writing suggests that the language experience of many pupils is concentrated in a relatively narrow range of types of writing.' (APU, 1987)

For this reason, the programmes of study and the statements of attainment in the ATs for both reading and writing stress the importance of a wide variety of text types. So, for example, the programmes of study for writing for children working towards key stage 1 (roughly those aged 5 to 8 years) specify that,

> Pupils should undertake a range of chronological writing including some at least of diaries, stories, letters, accounts of tasks they have done and of personal experiences, records of observations they have made, e.g. in a science or design activity, and instructions, e.g. recipes. [They should also] undertake a range of non-chronological writing which includes ... some at least of lists, captions, labels, invitations, greetings cards, notices, posters ... plans and diagrams, descriptions, e.g. of a person or place, and notes for an activity, e.g. in science or designing and making.

(DES, 1989; Cox, 1991)

There are two major reasons for this emphasis on a variety of text types, which continues through all four key stages of the curriculum. The first is the obvious one related to uses of literacy in everyday life: people need to be able to read safety warnings and to interpret railway timetables, to write reports and letters of complaint just as much as they need to be able to read and write stories and poems. The second reason is that different varieties of language have characteristically different linguistic features; this applies to vocabulary, to sentence syntax and to the overall organisation of the discourse. For example, nominal clauses are more likely to occur in personal narratives than in descriptions; relative clauses are particularly frequent in descriptions and explanations; adverbial clauses of condition often occur in instructions, and explanations; and so on. So pupils need to read different kinds of writing in order to meet the full range of grammatical structures in English; and they need to produce different kinds of writing so that they have plenty of opportunities to practise using these structures, since there is some evidence that there are certain grammatical forms that are first acquired through reading and writing and only later transferred to the spoken language repertoire (Perera, 1986). In other words, reading and writing are not just very useful practical skills; they are also powerful agents in the process of language development.

## Chronological and Non-chronological Writing

If teachers are to introduce their pupils to different varieties of writing in such a way that there is a structured and supportive progression from easier to harder kinds, then it is necessary to have a set of principles for the identification of text difficulty. The English Working Group (of which I was a member) formulated this set:

> Other things being equal, a writing task is easier if the organization is chronologi-
> cal; if the subject matter is drawn from personal experience; if the subject matter
> is concrete rather than abstract; and if the audience is known to the writer.'
>
> (DES, 1989; Cox, 1991)

I want to focus now solely on the question of chronological versus non-chronological organisation of a text.

The most obvious kind of chronological organisation is where a number of events or actions are presented in the order in which they occurred. A sequence of sentences, each with a dynamic verb in the simple past, will normally be interpreted as having an ordered temporal relationship. For example:

I got up.
I had a shower.
I had breakfast.
I got dressed.

The last three sentences could logically describe three actions which could happen in any order – they could simply be some of the things I did after getting up. But there is a strong likelihood that the linguistic sequence will be interpreted as reflecting the temporal sequence – and the inference will be drawn that I had breakfast in my dressing gown. The sense of temporal ordering can be reinforced by adverbials, e.g.

First, I had a shower.
Then, I had breakfast.
Next, I got dressed.

Or events can be presented out of sequence if a past perfect form of the verb is used, e.g.

I had breakfast.
I had already fed the cat.

where feeding the cat is clearly the earlier activity even though linguistically it follows the later activity of having breakfast. Such passages are chronologically organised (whether or not the events are presented in their order of occurrence) because the predominant relationship between the events is a temporal one. From the point of view of the reader, chronologically organised texts are easy to interpret at the level of the relationship between sentences, paragraphs and chapters because temporal sequence is a familiar and generally straightforward concept. (There may, of course, be linguistic or conceptual difficulty at sentence level.) By the same token, writers usually find the structuring of a piece that is susceptible to chronological organization unproblematic – you start at the beginning and present events in sequence until you come to the end. There is considerable evidence that children find it easier to write coherently about things that can be chronologically organised than about those that cannot (e.g. Wilkinson et al., 1979; Bereiter, 1980; Kantor & Rubin, 1981; Perera, 1984). The most obvious kind of chronologically organised text is the story, where we expect to start reading at the beginning and not to cheat by skipping to the last page to see how it ends. But non-fiction can also have a chronological organisation, e.g. biographies, reports, minutes of meetings, accounts of processes, etc. For instructions, such as workshop manuals, knitting patterns and cookery recipes, there is a very strict chronological requirement; we would be justifiably indignant if a recipe told us to slice the aubergines, fry them gently in olive oil, sprinkle them with grated cheese and brown them under a grill, and only then added that they should be sprinkled with salt and left to drain before being fried. Writing that is not organised chronologically may be structured in a wide variety of ways. For the reader this brings the problem of having to work out what the basis of the relationship is. This may have to be induced using common sense and knowledge of the subject matter, or it may be signalled linguistically by adverbials such as similarly (signalling a comparison), on the other hand (signalling a contrast), *therefore* (signalling a consequence), and so on. Unfortunately, several studies show that many pupils as old as 15, and with no language disorder, find these sentence connectives very difficult (e.g. Robertson, 1968; Gardner, 1977; Henderson, 1979). So the author writing textbooks for school children can either include connectives which they may not understand, or can leave the relationship implicit, which they may not be able to work out.

When pupils are themselves producing non-chronological writing they are faced with the problem of having to find the best way to organise their material. On the whole, an additive style of composing, where ideas are set down in the order in which they come into the writer's head, does not produce satisfactory non-chronological writing, as is clear from this extract from a piece by a 12-year-old girl:

> The Vikings were cruel and tortured their prisoners and they killed and slaughtered the mums and children. They poked them with spears and they were also very good craftsmen, for they carved their own boats and ships.
>
> (Burgess, 1973)

The programmes of study in the English curriculum are explicit about this organisational difficulty:

> Pupils should learn that, whereas chronological writing has a straightforward pattern of organisation, non-chronological types of writing can be organised in a variety of ways and so, generally, require more planning. By reading good examples of descriptions, explanations, opinions etc and by being given purposeful opportunities to write their own, they should be helped to plan and produce these more demanding types of writing.'
>
> (DES, 1989; Cox, 1991)

## Patterns of Organisation in Non-chronological Writing

If we look at non-fiction books written for children, we can see that they may be organised at a number of different levels and that the organisation is signalled in a variety of ways. Starting at the lowest level, sentences that share a common topic may be grouped into a paragraph. Paragraphs are commonly arranged in what I shall call a unit. In a great many non-fiction books produced for children up to about the age of 12, a unit is one double-page spread. I think the term 'unit' is preferable to the term 'chapter' because there is no normal expectation that chapters in a book will all be a uniform length or that they will always end at the foot of a right-hand page. Units may be grouped into sections or they may simply be compiled to make the book. Where there are sections they tend to be signalled visually by means of the typeface and layout; so a book on world religions, for example, has the three sections Beliefs, Worship, and Celebrations. These section headings are printed in capital letters between thin lines. Within each section there are from three to five units; for example, the section on celebrations contains units on Holy days, Family life, and Festivals. The unit titles are printed in lower case letters. Another book, on health education, has four sections, each containing either two or three units. In this case, each section heading is printed on a different background colour and the unit headings within the sections are also colour coded. So the section called Growing has a yellow background for the section heading and for the unit headings: Growing and changing, Year by year, and Looking ahead. This distinguishes the units from those in the Keeping Healthy section, for example, which have a pink background for their headings. It is obviously necessary for pupils to be aware of the significance of these details of presentation if they are to get the most from the book.

Sometimes sections and units are arranged in some logical order within the book; for example, a book on bridges starts with stepping stones, goes on to the simplest single arch bridge and then progresses through structures of increasing complexity, culminating in the cantilever bridge. But very often it would be possible for most of the sections or units to be rearranged without any effect on the meaning or comprehensibility of the whole. Indeed, this is reflected in the way teachers use the books, because it is perfectly possible in a book on Great Britain, say, to read the 12th unit, on London, before reading the 4th unit, on the monarchs of Britain, whereas darting round in this way in a work of fiction would be aberrant and unrewarding. To find patterns of organisation in non-chronological texts written for children, then, it is necessary to look at the structure of individual units and, particularly, of individual paragraphs.

Most often a unit begins with an introductory sentence that would read oddly if it was placed elsewhere. After that, though, it may well be the case that the four or five paragraphs that make up the unit have no relationship other than being on the same topic and could, therefore, have been printed in any order without any change of meaning. It is worth noticing how different this is from chronologically ordered writing, where changing the order of paragraphs is likely to make a significant change to the meaning. Where there is no sequential relationship between paragraphs, there is no dynamism within the text to carry the reader forward; this is just one factor that makes non-fiction generally harder to read than fiction of a similar measured level of reading difficulty.

Ideally, there should be a clear sense of an orderly relationship between sentences within a paragraph. This relationship can be of a number of different kinds; I shall illustrate some of the commonest with examples from non-fiction books written for primary-school children. There might be a general statement, followed by one or more illustrative examples, e.g 'There are many different ways of praying. People can say prayers out loud, or sing them, or say them silently to themselves.' Or the paragraph may begin with examples which are then drawn together in a general statement, e.g.'Keep Out! Caution! No Entry! are warnings. They tell you that a place isn't safe.'

The arrangement of sentences can reflect a spatial arrangement, as in this introduction to the geography of India, starting in the north and moving systematically southwards:'Some of the highest mountains in the world are in northern India. ... If you travel south from the mountains, you will come to a vast open plain. ... To the far west of the plains ... the cultivated fields eventually merge into the Thar Desert. The average rainfall in this desert region can be as little as 65 mm each year. To the east of the plains the rainfall is much heavier. ... Far to the south of the plains you will come to a wide plateau land, called the Deccan. Along the southern coasts, farmers harvest various types of palm trees for their oil.'

The relationship may be one of comparison, e.g.'Have you ever seen a dog lick a cut paw until it heals? When you cut your finger, you too need to keep it clean.'

Or it may be one of contrast, e.g.'Many people in India live simply. They do not have enough money to buy non-essential luxury goods. ...There are also some very rich people in India.'

A statement of a problem may be followed by its solution, e.g.'Railway locomotives are unable to climb steep hills. Therefore, bridges, tunnels and cuttings are used to keep the slope of the track as gentle as possible.'

Or the solution might come first, being followed by the problem it was intended to solve, e.g.'The Emperor Trajan ordered the building of this bridge over the River Tagus. The river was a major obstacle to troop movements.'

Similarly, in the cause–effect relationship, either may come first. Here the effect precedes the cause: 'Gandhi went to jail happily. He had made his point.' Whereas in the next example the cause comes first: 'Everyone's epidermis contains tiny amounts of dark colour called melanin. ... The more melanin your skin contains the darker its colour.'

These different relationships may be signalled linguistically by words such as *therefore, however, too, also,* for instance, but very often young readers are left to work out the relationship for themselves. For example, I was not immediately aware of the relationship between the following three paragraphs on first reading:

> 'People are very complicated and many things can make them different. They inherit how tall they are as adults, or the colour of their hair, from their parents and grandparents but other things are important too.
> 'People need a balanced diet. If they eat too much they can become fat and unhealthy. If they eat too little or the wrong sorts of food, they do not grow properly.'
> 'Children who live in different places grow up to know and understand different things. Some are used to hot places, others cold. Some live in towns, and others in the country...'

A moment's reflection tells us that the author is explaining that individual differences are caused by heredity, lifestyle and environment, but I feel that for young readers it would be helpful if the links between the ideas in the three paragraphs were marked more explicitly.

It is particularly unfortunate that it is sometimes the books for the very youngest readers that provide the least help in terms of organisation of the material. Here is an extract from a book on mice, in a series *(Macdonald Starters)* designed for infant children. There is a large full-colour picture on each page. The text is not divided into paragraphs or units but is simply a series of sentences that accompany the pictures.

> The spiny mouse has a tail which breaks easily.
> The pocket mouse has pouches in its cheeks.
> Sometimes there are too many mice.
> They eat everything they can find.
> These men are trying to poison mice.
> But the mice sometimes get used to poison.
> It does not kill them.
> Rats are like mice but much bigger.
> These rats live on a farm.
> Many rats live in towns.
> They are often dirty.
> They carry diseases.

> Scientists keep mice for experiments.
> This mouse has been taught to open a door.
> Mice were sent into space in rockets long before people.

In terms of its disjointedness, this extract (which consists entirely of contiguous sentences) reads startlingly like young children's attempts at non-chronological writing. The book starts misleadingly because it opens with a time, a place and some characters, so the first page sets up the expectation that a chronologically organised narrative will follow:

> It is the middle of the night.
> There are mice in the kitchen.

## Implications for the Classroom

This brief look at chronological and non-chronological writing suggests where some difficulties may lie and points to some ideas for overcoming them. As far as reading is concerned, it is helpful if teachers can take textual organisation into account as well as other factors such as vocabulary difficulty, interest level and so on when they are choosing books for young readers. Also, of course, it is important that teacher-produced worksheets should be as clearly structured as possible; when material can be presented in a chronological way, that provides a straightforward organising principle. I believe that pupils can be helped, too, to learn to recognise meaning relationships within a text. Teachers are used to providing reading activities that focus on word building and sentence meaning. I think it is rather less common to focus on patterns of organisation within a paragraph or unit. There are a number of activities that can help here. For example, pupils can be asked to provide sub-headings for each paragraph within a unit, or, if there are headings already, the teacher can photocopy the page, cut out the headings and get the children to match the headings to the text. If the sentences of a paragraph are typed out on separate lines, children can cut them up and give them to a partner to reassemble into a coherent whole. If the reconstituted version does not match the original, the pupils can discuss whether the meaning has been changed and which of the two orders they think is the better. Another possibility is to encourage children to highlight the structural words and phrases which signal relationships between sentences and paragraphs.

As far as writing is concerned, the first essential is that children have plenty of experience of reading well-organised non-chronological texts before they are expected to produce any of their own. If their non-fiction diet consists of books like the one above on mice, then it is not surprising if their writing is disjointed and incoherent. Another problem that book exemplifies is that many non-fiction texts are heavily dependent on pictures and illustrations. If children write in that style but without the accompanying pictures then their language will read rather oddly. We can make the comparison with chronological writing, where children hear and tell chronologically structured stories and accounts regularly and often, both inside and outside school.

Secondly, teachers need to recognise that non-chronological writing makes much heavier planning demands on the writer than chronological writing does. For pupils with language problems, this may well mean that the writing task should be reframed in such a way that it can be handled chronologically. But if this is not possible, it is a good idea to discuss the possible ways in which the material could be structured and then to provide a framework before the writing begins. For I am convinced that it is by recognising some of the linguistic and cognitive demands that are made upon pupils as they attempt to read and to write a variety of text types, that we can be in a position to provide the kind of support that is needed by all those who struggle to become literate.

## References

APU (1987). *Pupils' Attitudes to Writing*. London: HMSO.

BEREITER, C. (1980). Development in writing. In: Gregg, L.W. and Steinberg, E.R. (Eds), *Cognitive Processes in Writing*. Hillsdale, NJ: Lawrence Erlbaum and Associates.

BURGESS, C. (1973). *Understanding Children Writing* Harmondsworth: Penguin.

COX B. (1991). *Cox on Cox*. London: Hodder & Stoughton.

DES (1989). *English for Ages 5 to 16*. London: HMSO.

GARDNER, P.L. (1977). Logical connectives in science: a summary of the findings. Report to the Australia Education Research and Development Committee.

HENDERSON, I. (1979). *The use of connectives by fluent and not-so-fluent readers*. DEd. thesis, Columbia University Teachers' College.

KANTOR, K. J. and RUBIN, D. L. (1981). Between speaking and writing: processes of differentiation. In: Kroll, B.M. and Vann, R.J. (Eds): *Exploring Speaking Writing Relationships: Connections and Contrasts*. Urbana, IL: National Council of Teachers of English.

PERERA, K. (1984). *Children's Writing and Reading*. Oxford: Blackwell.

PERERA, K. (1986). Language acquisition and writing. In: Fletcher, P. and Garman, M. (Eds), *Language Acquisition* ,2nd edn. Cambridge: CUP.

ROBERTSON, J.E. (1968). Pupil understanding of connectives in reading. *Reading Research Quarterly* , 3, 387–417.

WILKINSON, A., BARNSLEY, G., HANNA, P. and SWAN, M. (1979). Assessing language development: the Crediton Project. *Language for Learning,* 1, 50–76.

# Chapter 15
# Promoting reading and spelling skills through speech therapy

JOY STACKHOUSE

## A Hidden Speech and Language Disorder?

Traditionally, it has not been considered that reading and spelling development and difficulties would be included in the everyday work of the developmental speech and language therapist. However, research has shown that children with spoken language difficulties present with written language problems and that those children who are most at risk for specific reading and spelling problems are those whose speech difficulty has no clear structural or neurological cause (Stackhouse, 1982; Bishop, 1985; Stackhouse, 1990).

Furthermore, there is increasing evidence that children with dyslexia may have associated subtle and persistent speech and language difficulties. In a recent paper, Stackhouse and Wells (1991) presented a case of an eleven year old boy with a reading age of 8;09 and a spelling age of 7;02 who had been referred for an assessment of his spoken and written language skills. Parents had become increasingly concerned about his poor progress in reading and spelling skills and noted that his speech could be 'unclear' at times. Richard had not been seen by a speech therapist before but there was a family history of dyslexic difficulties, word finding problems and poor memory.

A comprehensive psycholinguistic assessment revealed that Richard had a specific speech output deficit. He had word-finding difficulties, sound-processing problems and high-level speech difficulties. In contrast, he had normal speech-input skills, no difficulties with verbal comprehension and could express himself verbally using complex grammatical structures. These strengths had somewhat masked his other difficulties which were part and parcel of his reading and spelling problem.

Richard is a good example of how hidden speech and language difficulties may be manifested in poor literacy development and under-achievement at school. There seems to be an increasing number of children like Richard in mainstream schools. Some may have had speech therapy in the past, been discharged because of their improved intelligibility but continue to carry with them an underlying phonological disability. Others, like Richard, may never have been referred to speech therapy when young either because they were not considered to have a severe enough communication problem at the time or because this service was not available to them.

When the more subtle speech and language problems manifest in the form of reading and spelling problems later, subsequent investigations often focus on the symptoms of the learning problem rather than the underlying speech and language processing difficulties. This is where the speech and language therapist could have an important diagnostic role to play. Indeed, many of the associated problems found in children described as 'dyslexic'are also found in children with specific speech and language difficulties (Snowling, 1987). These include delayed speech and language development, persisting articulatory problems, word-finding problems, immature syntax development, perceptual, memory and sequencing difficulties, and trouble with segmentation and blending skills.

## Reading and Spelling Development

In order to understand this relationship between spoken and written language development and why a speech and language therapist might be involved in the educational process, it is necessary to examine the normal development of reading and spelling strategies. Frith (1985) has presented a three stage model of literacy development in which the child moves from an initial *logographic*, or visual, whole-word recognition strategy of reading, on to an *alphabetic* stage utilising letter–sound correspondences and finally into an *orthographic* phase dependent on segmentation of larger units: morphemes. In the first stage children's reading performance is limited by the extent of their orthographic lexicon, that is they can only read words that they know. Breakthrough to the alphabetic stage, however, allows them to tackle unfamiliar material since they can apply letter-sound rules. The final stage allows them to recognise larger chunks of words and therefore to read by analogy with known words more proficiently. Once the child has the skills to perform at each stage they can apply the most appropriate strategy for the task presented.

Spelling development moves through the same stages but not necessarily at exactly the same time. In fact, to begin with there is often a dissociation between reading and spelling development; children may be able to spell words that they cannot read and vice versa (Bradley and Bryant, 1979). However, if Frith's model is correct there should be a gradual increase in the application of letter-sound rules as their spelling develops.

A recent study attempted to track this development by examining children's spelling errors at different spelling ages (Stackhouse, 1989). Twenty-two children between the ages of 6;01 and 8;11 were divided into three groups on the basis of spelling age (range 5;11–13;06). Each child was asked to spell 30 words and the error data was analysed into three categories (after Ehri, 1985). The first error type – non-phonetic – involves no sound monitoring by the child (for example ORANGE spelt as oearasrie, or WASP as water) and is typical of the logographic stage of literacy development. The second – semiphonetic – indicates that the child is segmenting the target into its salient components but does not yet have sufficient letter knowledge or reading experience to know how to portray the bits in conventional print. Errors therefore include letter sounds and names used to represent syllables (for example bgul for BURGLAR, getr for GUITAR), and deletion of elements of clusters (for example bup for BUMP, soman for SNOWMAN). This primitive spelling does, however, mark a breakthrough to the alphabetic stage. The third category of spelling error is phonetic. As children increase their orthographic experience, they can present unfamiliar words sound by sound even though they have not yet learned the correct conventional spelling of the target. Such errors can be read back perfectly well and show proficient alphabetic spelling (for example bukit and spayd for BUCKET and SPADE).

The results revealed a steady increase of phonetic spellings with a marked decline of non-phonetic spellings around the spelling age of 7 years. In fact, non-phonetic spelling was never the predominant error type in even the beginner spellers. Rather, up until the spelling age of 8 semiphonetic spellings were most common. This significant trend in sound by sound spellings ($P < 0.05$) indicated that children do draw upon sound-processing skills in order to spell proficiently.

## Reading and Spelling Development in Speech-disordered Children

This development is in marked contrast to that found in speech-disordered children. In a longitudinal study, the reading and spelling skills of two speech-disordered children were investigated over a five-year period beginning when they were ten years old (Stackhouse, 1989). Both children were described as having developmental verbal dyspraxia – a motor programming speech disorder – and were being educated in a language unit attached to a normal school. In the following spellings of three syllable words you can see how Michael aged 11 is struggling over and over again to segment the bits in the words and in particular the clusters:

UMBRELLA – rberherrelrarlsrllles
CIGARETTE – satesatarhaelerari

Unfortunately, the more he tries to repeat the word the more inconsistent and distorted it becomes. Articulatory rehearsal can therefore not be used to support the segmentation of the target prior to it being spelt.

The second child, Caroline, aged 12 years, was also unable to use her speech output to aid sound segmentation of complex words. However, she had adopted a syllabic segmentation strategy as can be seen in her spelling by word components:

ADVENTURE – andbackself
REFRESHMENT – withfirstmint

Both of these children were found to have pervasive phonological deficits which interfered with their reading and spelling development. Even at the age of 15 their spelling errors were non-phonetic. They remained trapped in the logographic stage of literacy development and were unable to utilise alphabetic skills.

However, not all children seen by the speech and language therapist are as severe as Michael and Caroline. Many will be more like Richard discussed above, having subtle and well-hidden speech and language deficits. Moreover, not all of the children we should be concerned about will be at school. Indeed, much of the speech and language therapist's time may be devoted to younger children. It is in this group in particular that we should be able to identify the at risk child and have a prophylactic role. If children with specific reading and spelling problems have associated speech and language difficulties, then it follows that the future dyslexics are amongst the preschool children with speech and language problems. The speech and language therapist is therefore the first member of the education team to be able to initiate a preliteracy training programme. What activities would be helpful?

## Preliteracy Language Programme

Needless to say all of the activities involved in language enrichment programmes feed in to literacy development. In particular, lexical development and symbolic representations should be a focus. The speech and language therapist can help parents to select appropriate books for their language impaired child and ensure that book awareness is developing. This includes sequencing pictures of a story from left to right, abstracting the meaning from the context and engaging in 'pretend reading activities'. Technical skills are incorporated into this, such as holding the book the right way up and turning pages in the right order. Research has shown that children who are exposed to printed material in this way in the preschool years have an easier start at school and progress more quickly with their literacy development (Francis, 1982).

This general meta-language preparation enables the child to be ready to read logographically. In order to break through to the alphabetic stage of literacy development, however, the child needs to develop more specific alphabetic skills through increased phonological awareness.

## Phonological Awareness Training

Phonological awareness is a very broad term and refers to the child's ability to rhyme and to segment words into syllables and phonemes (Goswami and Bryant, 1990). In preschool children with delayed speech and language development, such phonological awareness training can be easily incorporated into nursery schools, language group work and speech therapy sessions as follows.

### Syllable Segmentation

Games involving musical instruments such as copying rhythms, identifying and producing the number of beats (i.e. syllables) in the children's names are popular preschool activities. This activity can be developed to suit older children. Richard mentioned above had difficulty detecting the number of syllables in multisyllabic words and this affected his spelling of them. 'Reading' visual morse code-type patterns and generating words of three or four syllables help the older child to focus on the syllable structure of the word before spelling it. This was in fact as far as Caroline had got in the examples given above.

Older language-disordered children will also need help at the morphophonological levels, for example, to understand that changing the position of the stressed beat in a word may change the meaning; compare RELAY versus RELAY, CONVERT versus CONVERT. Also, adding morphemes changes the phonology of the words, for example as in ELECTRIC, ELECTRICITY, ELECTRICIAN where the second letter C is pronounced as a 'k', 's' or 'sh' respectively. When spelling, adding morphemes may result in the addition (e.g. confer/conferring) or deletion (e.g. have/having) of graphemes. Mastery of these rules is characteristic of the orthographic stage of literacy development. Children with dyspraxic speech difficulties, however, find this problematic since speech errors disrupt the syllable structure of the word and this interferes with their reading and spelling performance.

## Rhyme

Rhyming ability correlates with literacy development and yet it is well known that speech and language disordered children have problems with learning to rhyme. Both Michael and Caroline performed poorly on rhyme production tasks. At the age of 11 Michael was still producing alliterative and semantic associations as rhyme responses; for example when asked 'What rhymes with iron?' he replied 'cannonballs'!

Testing rhyming skills is difficult in preschool children. Even though they may have some rhyming ability, they may fail to perform well on a rhyme test because they do not understand the instructions or what is expected of them. A starting point in assessment and therapy is therefore to examine the child's knowledge of popular nursery rhymes. The existence of such knowledge or the progress made with teaching nursery rhymes could be important prognostic factors for the development of other phonological skills and later reading ability (Maclean, Bryant and Bradley, 1988). However, this tacit awareness of rhyme needs to become more explicit if it is to be applied usefully to the literacy situation. In order to have a more conscious control over the manipulation of words, the child needs to be aware at some level that syllables can be divided up into an *onset*, that is everything preceding the vowel, and a *rime* – the remainder of the syllable. The following words all have different onsets but the same rime: C-AT, M-AT, FL-AT, SPR-AT.

Various activities can be carried out in the nursery class/language group to promote rhyme awareness. For example, nursery teachers have a large repertoire of rhyming action games. The speech and language therapist and the nursery teacher need to examine these activities together and incorporate them into programmes for language-delayed children. They can be supplemented by games such as 'Guess what I'm hiding?' or 'I went shopping and I bought ——' where semantic and rhyming clues are given, and by making up a rhyme corner or wall charts. More structured activities can be designed for individual children; such as finding rhyming objects hidden in pictures; older children can spot the odd one out in a series of auditorily presented words, for example BUN DOG FUN SUN (Bradley, 1980). Children who find this difficult should be encouraged to spot onset/rime pattern differences in the printed words. Gradually words where the grapheme pattern interferes with this are introduced, to push the child to abstract the auditory rhyme from the printed words, for example 'spot the odd one out in the printed series SEW GO NEW'.

## Phoneme Segmentation

Finally, games to promote phoneme segmentation are particulary helpful to the child beginning school. Although I-spy activities are often the
first to spring to mind, it is important to programme such activities from
easy to hard (Lewkowicz, 1980). At first, this may involve asking the child
closed questions such as 'Does CAR begin with /k/? – Yes or No?' The
next step may be to offer a forced alternative 'Does CAR begin with /k/ or
/z/.' This could then be followed by an open question 'What does CAR
begin with?' Children needing help with the sequencing of sounds might
be asked 'Does CAT begin with /k/ or /t/?' both sounds being in the word
but in different positions. As the child progresses more complex comparative awareness exercises can be given, such as 'Does CAR begin with the
same sound as CAN or ZOO?'. Where there is an articulatory difficulty,
the child's target/error sounds can be included in these activities.

## Phonological Awareness Training for Children with Speech and Language Disorders

Of course speech and language therapists have always worked on
phonological awareness training in their articulation therapy. However,
the aim of this therapy has been to increase intelligibility rather than promote reading and spelling skills. The Metaphon programme in particular
is an excellent example of phonological awareness training for young
children with speech and language delay (Howell and Dean, 1991). It
focuses their attention on the properties of sounds and on different
positions within the word. Contrasting sounds in minimal pairs, for
example tea/key/sea, increases the child's awareness of the onset/rime
structure of the syllable.

However, many of our routine activities fall short of making the
child's phonological awareness explicit enough to promote their literacy
development. Traditionally, speech and language therapists have focused
on the auditory–vocal channel with our preschool children and ignored
the visual stimuli of the printed letter. In a longitudinal study, Bradley
and Bryant (1983) have shown the importance of linking phonological
awareness training with the printed form. A group of 6-year-old children
whose training in rhyme and alliteration was coupled with the presentation of plastic letters showing how each sound was represented and seg-
mented had made more progress with their literacy development when
followed up 2 years later than children who received phonological
awareness training alone. Both of these groups, however, made more
progress than the two control groups; one of which received training in
semantic classification only and the other had received no training at all.

Children with more serious speech and language difficulties will need continued multisensory training to develop both their spoken and written language skills. Adding the grapheme alone may not be sufficient. Younger children may benefit from the Letterland Scheme *. Here letters are associated with characters which are easily remembered, for example Bouncing Benjamin Bunny, Clever Cat, and the Hairy Hat Man. Articulation and phonological therapy linked with the printed word can be carried out using these symbols. These are preferred to the sound symbol pictures traditionally used in articulation therapy, which may not be phoneme–grapheme matched; for example the rabbit representing /f/, the candle for /p/ or the jelly for /m/. Although these may be quite fun for younger children, their use in more explicit phonological awareness tasks is limited and teachers have commented on their inappropriateness.

Another useful teaching tool in speech and literacy, training is colour coding. The Edith Norrie Letter Case provides some useful material†. Letter cards are colour coded; vowels are red, and voiced and voiceless consonants are green and black. The letters are then organised in a tray dependent on their place of articulation; front/middle/back. Children who find segmentation of multisyllabic words difficult are aided by knowing that they need to have regular splashes of red in a sequence of letters.

Speech and language therapists may however want to make the articulatory cueing even more explicit. This can be done by using colour to remind the child of the manner of the sounds, for example all fricative sounds in green (f z sh); while diacritics can be used to show place of articulation, for example lips drawn under all bilabial sounds (p b m). A voicing symbol can be placed over all voiced sounds (Stackhouse, 1985). Alternatively, or additionally, a motor gesture can be used as an articulatory reminder as in Cued Articulation‡. The therapist can mix and match the cues to suit the child; the aim being that the child is improving his intelligibility, phonological awareness and literacy skills simultaneously by focusing on the interaction of auditory, articulatory and visual feedback.

## Summary

Table 15.1 shows the metalinguistic and linguistic prerequisites for each stage of literacy development. The left-hand column lists the stages of literacy development; the right-hand column shows what back-up skills are required in order for a child to move on to the next stage of literacy development.

This paper has focused on phonological awareness skills in particular. The development of phonological awareness is a gradual and complex process dependent on the coming together of acoustic, articulatory and

*Further information from Letterland Ltd, Barton, Cambridge, England, CB3 7AY.
†Available from The Helen Arkell Dyslexia Centre, 14 Crondace Road, London, SW6.
‡Futher information from ICAN, 10 Bowling Green Lane, Farringdon, London, EC1.

**Table 15.1** The metalinguistic and linguistic prerequistes for each stage of literacy development

| Stages of literacy development | Metalinguistic and linguistic development |
|---|---|
| Preliterate | Speech/language development |
| | Symbolic representations |
| | Communication skills |
| Logographic | Interest in print |
| | Pretended reading/writing |
| Alphabetic | Phonological awareness |
| | Articulatory skills |
| | Alphabetic knowledge |
| | Orthographic experience |
| Orthographic | Morphophonology |

orthographic information. Children with written and spoken language difficulties have poor phonological awareness and require specific help through multisensory remediation programmes.

## Conclusion

The speech and language therapist is well equipped to investigate and develop back-up skills that children require in order to progress with their literacy development. There are a number of ways in which activities originally designed to improve spoken language can be extended to promote written language. The speech and language therapist, however, is not trained to teach reading and spelling (unless they have gone on to specialise post qualification); for this expertise we must look to the teacher. Once the child is at school, the therapist and teacher have an important collaborative role in integrating the spoken and written language programmes.

## References

BISHOP, D.V.M. (1985). Spelling ability in congenital dysarthria: evidence against articulatory coding in translating between phonemes and graphemes. *Cognitive Neuropsychology*, 2, 229–251.

BRADLEY, L. (1980). *Assessing Reading Difficulties*. London: MacMillan Educational.

BRADLEY, L. and BRYANT, P. (1979). Independence of reading and spelling in backward and normal readers. *Developmental Medicine and Child Neurology*, 21, 504–514.

BRADLEY, L. and BRYANT, P. (1983). Categorising sounds and learning to read: a causal connexion. *Nature*, 301, 419.

EHRI, L.C. (1985). Sources of difficulty in learning to spell and read. In: Wolraich, M.L., and Routh, D. (Eds), *Advances in Developmental and Behaviourial Paediatrics*. Greenwich, CT: Jai Press.

FRANCIS, H. (1982). *Learning to Read – Literate Behaviour and Orthographic Knowledge*. London: Unwin Education.

FRITH, U. (1985). Beneath the surface of developmental dyslexia. In: Patterson, K.E., Marshall, J.C. and Coltheart, M. (Eds), *Surface Dyslexia*. London: Routledge and Kegan Paul.

GOSWAMI, U. and BRYANT, P. (1990). *Phonological Skills and Learning To Read*. Hillsdale, NJ: Lawrence Erlbaum Associates Ltd.

HOWELL, J. and DEAN, E. (1991). *Treating Phonological Disorders in Children*. Kibworth: Far Communications.

LEWKOWICZ, N.K. (1980). Phonemic awareness training: What to teach and how to teach it. *Journal of Educational Psychology*, 72, 686–700.

MACLEAN, M., BRYANT, P. and BRADLEY, L. (1988). Rhymes, nursery rhymes and reading in early childhood. In: Stanovich, K.E. (Ed.), *Children's Reading and the Development of Phonological Awareness*, pp. 11–37. Detroit: Wayne State University Press.

SNOWLING, M. (1987). *Dyslexia. A Cognitive Developmental Perspective*. Oxford: Basil Blackwell.

STACKHOUSE, J. (1982). An investigation of reading and spelling performance in speech disordered children. *British Journal of Disorders of Communication*, 17, 53–60.

STACKHOUSE, J. (1985). Segmentation, speech and spelling difficulties. In: Snowling, M. (Ed.), *Children's Written Language Difficulties*, pp. 96–115. NFER-Nelson.

STACKHOUSE, J. (1989). *Phonological dyslexia in children with developmental verbal dyspraxia*. Unpublished PhD Thesis, Psychology Department, University College London.

STACKHOUSE, J. (1990). Phonological deficits in developmental reading and spelling disorders. In: Grunwell, P.(Ed.), *Developmental Speech Disorders*, pp. 163–182. Edinburgh: Churchill-Livingstone.

STACKHOUSE, J. and WELLS, B. (1991). Dyslexia: The obvious and hidden speech and language disorder. In: Snowling, M. and Thomson, M. (Eds), *Dyslexia. Integrating Theory and Practice*. London: Whurr.

# Chapter 16
# Collaboration between speech and language therapists and teachers

JANNET A. WRIGHT

## Introduction

The research described in this chapter was an attempt to discover and describe current patterns of collaboration between teachers and therapists. Therapists were asked to say why they believed such collaboration was important and to identify factors which they felt facilitated successful collaboration between themselves and teachers.

During their undergraduate training speech and language therapists are expected to acquire knowledge, skills and attitudes that enable them to work with both adults and children who have communication problems. They study both the theory and management of children with language impairment. When working in the clinic they already try to involve the family in the therapeutic process, as much as possible, as recommended by writers such as Cooper, Moodley and Reynell (1978) and McConkey (1985). If the student is working clinically in a paediatric hospital department or community health centre, there are many opportunities to meet and involve a family in the speech therapy process, although a special arrangement may have to be made to visit a school to see a child and class teacher. If, however, the students are working in language units or special schools, where their supervising therapist is based, it is often harder to involve the rest of the family as the children may live some distance from that centre. But in these settings the therapist is at least on the same site as the child's teacher, and it is the contact between these two professionals which is of interest in this chapter.

In the last few years more speech and language therapy students have found themselves accompanying their clinician into mainstream schools while they are on clinical placement. Increasing numbers of qualified therapists are devising their own models of collaboration for working in schools because in some authorities therapists are spending a great deal of time in mainstream schools, either as a result of district policy or through specifically created posts to support children with statements. These models are beginning to be published, enabling other practitioners to use them or adapt them to their own working environment (Whitehouse, Beazley and Jones, 1987; Newman and Elks, 1990; Stockbridge and Upchurch, 1990; Harries and Martin; 1990).The data in this paper were collected before these models began to appear but it is hoped that the details will provide a useful starting point for those who are developing such models, as well as useful background information.

## Why Should Speech and Language Therapists and Teachers try to Collaborate ?

A child with a poorly developed or limited linguistic system can present the class teacher with a challenge. For example, classroom instructions may be missed due to inattention or the child may be socially immature because of the language difficulties and so may become isolated from peers. A language disability or communication problem may co-exist with other physical or cognitive problems. In fact, for some children, these other difficulties may be a contributing factor to a language disability. Children who are identified as having language difficulties are at risk of failure in an educational setting (Hall and Tomblin, 1978; Drillien and Drummond, 1983; Aram, Ekelman and Nation, 1984). Bishop and Edmundson (1987) found that the children in their study who still had language problems at 5;6 years also had difficulty with reading comprehension, spoken language skills and some non-verbal tasks.The introduction of speaking and listening as Attainment targets in English (DES, 1988) should lead to an increased awareness and concern about children who have communication problems.

Involving the class teacher when a child has a communication problem will help that individual child receive coordinated therapeutic and educational support. Meyers, Parsons and Martin (1979) suggest other reasons why speech and language therapists and teachers might want to work together. These include the large numbers of clients who are not seen or offered help by the present service organisation, a move from direct service delivery to indirect service delivery, and a continual demand for more therapists.

There is also a wide variation in the way speech and language therapy services are delivered; until recently they were the responsibility of individual District Speech Therapy Managers and consequently the policies in one district health authority varied considerably from those in an adjacent authority or between rural and urban areas. The variety in service delivery is reflected in the way the service is provided for children with communication problems who are attending a nursery or a school. Speech and language therapists may be based in a health centre, responsible for the therapy offered to a large number of nurseries and schools, or they may be based in a school or a unit attached to a school, for a specific number of sessions a week. Language units or special schools may have therapists assigned full-time to them or the therapy is provided on a part-time basis by one or more therapists. The children who are helped by both therapists and teachers are receiving a 'multi-professional' approach, but this is not easy as the DES Circular 22/89 acknowledges 'Effective multi-professional work requires cooperation, collaboration and mutual support on the part of the contributors' DES (1989).

The child with a communication problem may be the concern of many different professionals. However, teachers and speech and language therapists are often significant figures for the language impaired school-age child. In England and Wales these two professional groups are mainly employed by education and health authorities respectively. They go through a different training and work within different organisational systems but are expected to collaborate in order to help children with communication problems.

### What is Collaboration?

Collaboration is the joining together of 2 or more individuals in an egalitarian relationship to achieve a mutually determined goal

Conoley and Conoley (1982)

The egalitarian nature is the most distinguishing characteristic of collaborative strategy. Collaborative strategy joins the consultant and consultee in the determination of the goals, problem definitions and solution set

Caplan (1976)

Collaboration between people, who are members of different professional groups, requires effort from both sides. Johnson, Pugach and Devlin (1990) believe that both teachers and therapists have to recognise the limits of their training and their own professional biases in order to collaborate effectively. However, some colleagues fear that a move towards collaboration will take them away from face-to-face contact with the client. Conoley (1981) acknowledges that some professionals believe that one must be in direct contact with the 'pathology' and Frassineli, Superior and Meyers (1983) put forward the view that some therapists have an 'ingrained disposition towards direct therapy'.

It is not intended to suggest that every speech and language therapist has to work in a similar way. However, when one works with people who have communication problems, it will be necessary to 'collaborate' at some point with either other professionals or relatives. The egalitarian aspect of collaboration is difficult to achieve if a therapist has been asked to see a child in school and give an 'expert' opinion; it is easier to achieve where the close proximity and familiarity of teacher and therapist in a particular school, can facilitate a working partnership (Thomas, 1987; Miller, 1989). This proximity can reduce intergroup conflict as Pettigrew (1986) states when talking about the Contact Hypothesis. However, many factors can interfere with a successful partnership, such as lack of support from the head, size of school population, number of staff and timetabling arrangements and a lack of motivation.

## The Study

In order to discover whether speech and language therapists thought collaboration was important and how they went about it, a survey was carried out in England and Wales. The data described in this chapter were collected using a postal questionnaire. This method was chosen because it is useful with a specific professional group where the topic explored, via the questionnaire, is of particular interest to the members of that group (Moser and Kalton, 1971).

Speech and language therapists working in Scotland, Northern Ireland and for the British Forces in Germany were excluded from the survey; as were therapists working in the private sector or employed by organisations outside the National Health Service. This was because their terms of employment and the structure of the health service and educational organisation in which they work are significantly different from those of their colleagues in the National Health Service.

An initial letter was sent to 97 District Speech Therapy Managers (DSTMs). The response was enthusiastic; 75 wrote positive replies providing their support for this venture. These managers were sent copies of the questionnaires and they were asked to hand these out to their staff who were based in clinics or unit/school. Contact was made with speech therapists via their managers because first it was hoped that support from management would increase the rate of return and secondly, although encouraged to join, not every practising therapist is a member of the professional body, the College of Speech and Language Therapists. DSTMs are likely to employ both members and non-members. Contact with therapists through their manager hopefully would produce a representative sample.

Therapists who were health centre based and those who were unit/school based were identified as two separate groups. Over all 756 questionnaires were sent out; 459 were returned. This was a response rate of 61%. After rejecting inappropriate or spoiled questionnaires the final number of returns analysed was 443 Of these, 235 were from clinic-based therapists and 208 from school-based therapists.

## Description of Sample Population

*Clinic-based Therapists.* Those who work in a clinical setting were asked to indicate where their clinic was based, for example, hospital department, health centre, assessment centre or any other base. A Community Health Clinic was the base for 88% (206) of the respondents. Here therapists see clients and carry out administrative duties.In this group. on average, the therapists had been practising for 8 years; 43% had 3 years experience or less and 57% had more than 3 years. Some had as many as 37 years experience. In spite of this only 29% of them felt that they were specialist therapists. All these characteristics indicated that contact had been made with an appropriate group of clinic-based therapists.

*School-based Therapists.* The therapists in this group were based in schools or units, 144 of them worked as the only therapist in such a setting. The educational settings that they were in included language units, schools for children with physical problems, moderate and severe learning difficulties, autism and sensory deficits. In this group, on average, the therapists had been practising for 9 years; 28% had 3 years experience or less and 72% had more than 3 years experience.

## Contact Between Therapists and Teachers

Therapists who work in a school or a unit are on the same site as the teachers that they need to talk to.They do not have to make a special journey to see a class teacher, as the clinic-based therapist does. Thus the first contact between a therapist from a health centre and a teacher is very important in establishing a future pattern of collaboration. In a school the first contact between teacher and therapist does not carry the same significance. In school such a discussion may be timetabled. Information about these first contacts and meetings in school is given below.

*School-based Therapists.* It might be assumed that in a school or unit many teachers and therapists would have their meetings timetabled, indicating the importance placed on a sharing of information. In fact only 25% of the school-based therapists said that their meetings were timetabled. The 75% who did not have time allocated in this way said that their discussions took place in the non-teaching time. Break time and lunch time were the most popular times, followed by the time after school. The time spent in such discussions was on average up to 15 minutes, which 53% of the respondents felt was sufficient. The period before school began was rarely used for discussion between these two professional groups. The most popular venue for discussion was a separate room, possibly the staff room, followed by a classroom without any children in it. At times the discussion took place in a classroom while the children were present and occasionally in a corridor.

*Clinic-based Therapists.* It is more complicated for a clinic-based therapist than a school-based colleague to make contact with a teacher; a teacher is only available to come to the telephone at certain times in the school day and these times may not coincide with the therapist's proximity to a phone. If the view is taken that contact will be hard to make, then it is important to know if the initial flow of information between teacher and therapist, school and clinic, is part of an established routine. To discover the answer to this question, the therapists were asked if they made initial routine contact with a teacher when a child they were asked to see attended a nursery or school. It was acknowledged that such contact may be by telephone, letter or face-to-face. Out of the 232 therapists who replied to this question 62% (144) said they did make initial contact as a matter of routine, while 38% (88) did not. The fact that over a third of the respondents did not make contact as a matter of course causes some concern, because without such contact the teacher may not be aware of the possibility of educational problems that can be associated with language disability. It also raises questions about how the therapist views the teacher's role in facilitating language development within the classroom as well as the teacher's role with a child who has specific language problems. If initial contact is not made and the teacher is not aware that a child is about to start speech and language therapy, it is difficult for a working partnership to develop.

Therapists may decide, with parental permission, to make a visit to the school to meet the class teacher and see the child using their language skills in a different setting. This often means a special journey for the therapists and, as few schools are able to cover for the class teacher, special arrangements in the school. However, 95% of the clinic-based therapists stated that they were able to talk to the class teacher that they wanted to when they visited the school, although they did have to fit into the teacher's timetable. The time spent in discussion on this first visit was between 10 and 60 min, which the majority of respondents felt was sufficient time. Subsequent visits to the same school were usually no more than 25 min in length, in fact a time span of 5–15 min seemed most popular. If the therapist was visiting a nursery school or class this discussion most frequently took place in the classroom with children present. This is not the easiest situation in which to concentrate and exchange important information. However, for children of 5 years and older the staff room or another separate room was the most common venue. The second choice was the classroom but without the children.

### Therapists who have Worked Closely with Teachers

Of the school-based therapists who replied 92% said that they had worked closely with at least one teacher, whereas only 72% of the clinic-based therapists had worked closely with at least one teacher. This was usually the child's class teacher, although sometimes a particular teacher had sought help from the therapist or had shown a special interest in language. The therapists were asked to think of a recent case where they had worked with a teacher and to indicate who carried out the assessment of a child's speech and language, who planned the therapy and who carried out the intervention. The people who may be involved in this process included the teacher, the therapist, both of them, a nursery nurse, or non-teaching classroom assistant.

*Assessment.* Both the clinic-based therapists and the school-based therapists reported very little joint assessment. The clinic-based therapists did not indicate that the teacher was involved at all but it was more surprising to find that only a small number of school-based therapists mentioned the teacher as a partner in the assessment procedure.

*Planning.* In this area there was a marked distinction between the two groups of therapists. Half of the school-based therapists who answered this question, reported that they planned the intervention with the teacher, but only a third of the clinic-based therapists shared the planning with the teacher.

*Intervention.* The responses from both the school-based and the clinic-based therapists, showed that any intervention was most likely to be offered as a combination of some group work and some individual work. This occurred most frequently outside the classroom. The school-based therapists did work more frequently in the classroom than the clinic-based therapists but still were inclined to withdraw the child from the classroom for most of the time. Both groups answered that a joint approach, where the therapist and the teacher carried out the therapy, was common. However, if only one adult was going to carry out the therapy it was most likely to be the therapist. The fact that it was common for both the teacher and therapist to carry out the intervention but that the child was assessed by the therapist and the therapy was planned by the therapist, raises the question of how involved or committed to a piece of work the teacher may feel if they had no involvement in the planning. It can then be difficult to remember to carry out the intervention and maintain the work as a priority. As one respondent wrote: 'teachers and therapists both need to understand why they're doing what they're doing.'

## Why do Therapists Think Collaboration is Important ?

In the second section of the questionnaire both groups of therapists were asked to respond to a number of open questions. These responses were then analysed using a qualitative approach adapted from Miles and Huberman (1984).The replies were analysed for common features and these features were then coded in order to highlight and extract the common information. There were very few respondents from either group who did not think collaboration was a good thing. The reasons they gave included a belief that both professionals had or should have the same goals, that it was important to pool information, and that collaboration ensured an effective outcome for the child. Their responses also indicated an awareness of increased job satisfaction and of helping professional development. They also perceived an increase in the level of parental satisfaction.

## Perception of Teachers' Roles with Language-impaired Children

The speech therapists saw teachers as having certain roles/functions in facilitating a child's language development generally as well as being involved in specific work on language disorders. The role of the teacher with language impaired children was further explored when therapists were asked to identify the skills and knowledge that they believed teachers had in order to work effectively with these children. Speech and language therapists'perceptions of teachers' skills and knowledge and their assumptions about what teachers can do were described in some detail in response to this question. The comments could be grouped under the following areas. They believed that teachers had:

1. General knowledge about a child's development.
2. Specific knowledge about a child's performance in certain areas.

3. Specialist teaching skills.
4. A constant point of reference provided by the child's peer group in the class.

The therapists recognised that children behave in different ways in a variety of settings and class teachers are in a position to observe more of this variable behaviour than they are.

*Factors which Facilitate Collaboration*

Both groups of therapists were asked to identify the factors which encouraged collaboration. There was considerable agreement between the school-based and the clinic-based therapists about this. They believed that mutual goals were an important motivation factor in the collaboration process. The issue of 'time' was raised by the majority of respondents. They usually specified what they needed this time for: for example discussion, joint planning and evaluation of progress. Many felt that it was important in facilitating collaboration to appreciate each other's particular professional knowledge and contribution to the working partnership. Regular contact between therapist and teacher was seen as a crucial factor. For some the perceived level of management support was seen as an important issue.

To summarise, it appears that mutual goals can provide the motivation for members of two different professional groups to make the time for regular contact.

**Conclusion**

The two groups of therapists showed some predicted and some unpredicted responses to the questionnaire. A higher proportion of school-based therapists than clinic based therapists had worked closely with teachers. The fact that so many clinic-based therapists had worked with teachers was a surprise, especially as teachers were not always contacted as a matter of routine. The length of time clinic-based therapists spent on subsequent visits was quite short. This does not seem enough time to discuss progress in any detail but perhaps this was not the important point. These visits afforded the opportunity for a more regular contact between the two professionals which was felt to be important to facilitate collaboration.

The school-based therapists did collaborate more than the clinic-based therapists but there was still a high proportion of assessment and planning of programmes which was done only by the therapist. As many of the speech therapy sessions took place outside the classroom there needs to be some discussion time so that the therapist and teacher can exchange information and ideas on how to help a child. However very, few school-based therapists had discussion time scheduled, so this had to be worked into the school day on an *ad hoc* basis.The curriculum was not explicitly mentioned as a vehicle to facilitate collaboration, but may have been subsumed under the term 'common goals'.

The two groups had similar ideas about the reasons for collaboration and what facilitated it, but their responses indicate that collaboration is not actually taking place. There is evidence that some therapists are working with or alongside teachers, but this needs to be developed.The next stage in this study is to interview both teachers and therapists to analyse the process of collaboration in more detail.The answers to these questions will, we hope, help us to educate our speech therapy students to work collaboratively with teachers.

## References

ARAM, D.M., EKELMAN, B.L. and NATION, J.E. (1984).Preschoolers with language disorders: 10 years later. *Journal of Speech and Hearing Research,* 27, 232–244.

BISHOP, D.V.M. and EDMUNDSON, A. (1987). Specific language impairment as a maturational lag : evidence from longitudinal data on language and motor development. *Developmental Medicine and Child Neurology,* 29, 442–459.

CAPLAN, G.(1976). *The Theory and Practice of Mental Health Consultation.* London: Tavistock Publications.

CONOLEY, J.C. (Ed.) (1981). *Consultation in Schools : Theory Research Procedures.* London: Academic Press.

CONOLEY, J.C. and CONOLEY, C.W. (1982). *School Consultation : A Guide to Practice and Training.*Oxford: Pergamon.

COOPER, J., MOODLEY, M. and REYNELL, J. (1978). *Helping Language Development.* London: Edward Arnold.

DES (1988). *The Education Reform Act.* London: HMSO.

DES (1989). *Assessment and Statements of Special Educational Need Procedures within the Education, Health and Social Services.* Circular 22/89. London: HMSO.

DRILLIEN, C. and DRUMMOND, M. (1983). *Development Screening and the Child with Special Needs. Spastics International Medical Publications.* London: Heinemann.

FRASSINELLI, L., SUPERIOR, K. and MEYERS, J. (1983). *A Consultation Model for Speech and Language Interaction.* Rockville, MD: American Speech, Language and Hearing Association.

HALL, PK. and TOMBLIN, J.B. (1978). A follow-up study of children with articulation and language disorders. *Journal of Speech and Hearing Disorders,* 43, 227–241.

HARRIES, G.and MARTIN, S.(1990). Developing good practice together. In: Wright, J. and Kersner, M. (Eds), *Working Together for Children with Communication Problems, Proceedings of a Study Day,* pp. 71–75. NHCSS.

JOHNSON, L.J., PUGACH, M.C. and DEVLIN, S. (1990). Professional collaboration. *Teaching Exceptional Children,* Winter 1990.

MCCONKEY, R. (1985). *Working with Parents. A Practical Guide for Teachers and Therapists*. London: Croom Helm.

MEYERS, J., PARSONS, R.D. and MARTIN, R. (1979). *Mental Health Consultation in the Schools*. San Francisco: Jossey-Bass Publishers.

MILES, M.B. and HUBERMAN, A.M. (1984). *Qualitative Data Analysis: A Sourcebook of New Methods*. London: Sage.

MILLER, L. (1989). Classroom-based language intervention. *Language, Speech and Hearing Services in Schools*, 20 ,149–152.

MOSER, C.A. and KALTON, G. (1971). *Survey Methods in Social Investigation*. London: Heineman.

NEWMAN, S. and ELKS, E. (1990). Speech therapists and teachers : exploring systematic joint practice for the child with a communication disorder. In: Wright, J. and Kersner, M. (Eds),*Working Together for Children with Communication Problems, Proceedings of a Study Day*, pp. 76–94. NHCSS.

PETTIGREW, T.F. (1986). The intergroup contact hypotheses reconsidered. In: Hewston, M. and Brown, R. (Eds), *Contact and Conflict in Intergroup Encounters*. Oxford: Basil Blackwell.

STOCKBRIDGE, G. and UPCHURCH, M. (1990). Two Way Talk. In: Wright, J. and Kersner, M. (Eds), *Working Together for Children with Communication Problems. Proceedings of a Study Day*, pp. 95–105. NHCSS.

THOMAS, G. (1987). Extra people in the primary classroom. *Educational Research*, 29, 173–181

WHITEHOUSE, J.,BEAZLEY, S. and JONES, H. (1987). Establishing Partnership between Speech Therapists and Teachers involved with hearing-impaired children. In: *The Proceedings of the 9th Annual Conference of the College of Speech Therapists*. London: College of Speech Therapists.

# Chapter 17
# Principled decision making in the remediation of children with phonological disorders

PAMELA GRUNWELL

## Introdution

The focus of this chapter is best introduced by examining the three key terms in the title. In seeking to establish principles of decision making in clinical practice, one is trying to delineate a set of guidelines whereby the clinician can identify explicitly, justifiably and confidently treatment goals and priorities. The planning of remediation involves, in this paper, the identification of the initial treatment programme and the monitoring and modification of that programme throughout its implementation. The treatment of children with phonological disorders is a major aspect of many speech and language therapists' case load.

The term 'developmental phonological disorder' or 'phonological disability' is customarily used to refer to children with a specific language learning disability affecting speech production when their language difficulties cannot be attributed to known and detectable aetiological factors such as general learning disability, intellectual deficit, neuro-motor disorder, psychiatric disturbance or environmental factors. The classic clinical characteristics of these children are:

1. Almost completely unintelligible spontaneous speech resulting primarily from consonant deviations from adult target pronunciations.
2. Over 4 years of age, i.e. past the age at which speech is normally intelligible to persons from outside the child's immediate social envirment. When children are developing language normally, by 4;0–4;6 the target phonological system has been largely acquired.
3. Normal hearing for speech.

4. No anatomical or physiological abnormalities of the speech producing mechanism.
5. No detectable neurological dysfunction relevant to speech production.
6. Intellectual abilities adequate for the development of spoken language through the normal socialisation process.
7. Comprehension of spoken language appropriate (at least) to mental age.
8. Apparently adequate expressive language abilities in terms of range of vocabulary and utterance length (this latter presumably reflecting syntactic structures of some complexity, which usually cannot be accurately assessed because of the unintelligibility of the speech).
(See Gibbon and Grunwell, 1990 for the latest restatement of these characteristics.)

Clinical experience and research indicate that the occurrence of the condition in its pure classical form is rare (Shriberg et al., 1986; Gibbon and Grunwell, 1990). An appreciable number of children presenting with this type of speech disorder have a history of hearing problems of a mild nature, e.g. otitis media with effusion. Many of the children have detectable cognitive–linguistic deficits in both comprehension and production. Their educational progress is often slow and they may exhibit attention problems. In addition, as indicated in other chapters in this volume, there is frequent evidence of familial history of language problems. It is for these children across this broad range that the principles and procedures described in this chapter have been primarily developed.

Notwithstanding this central focus, these approaches are applicable in the treatment of children with other types of speech disorders. The speech production patterns associated with an identifiable handicapping condition (or 'organic disorder') often have phonological consequences; for example the backing pattern in which /t d/ are realised as [k g] in cleft palate speech (Grunwell, 1988; Ingram, 1989). A phonological orientation to treatment may be appropriate alongside articulatory training in such an instance. In addition, there may be developmental dimensions to the mispronunciations in the patterns of speech of children with organic disabilities. These will require investigation and intervention within a phonological framework (Grunwell, 1990).

## Basis for Decision Making

The basis upon which decisions in treatment planning are made is a phonological assessment and evaluation. It is essential that the phonological assessment employed reveal the characteristics of the pronunciation disorder. The assessment findings must provide answers to the questions posed in the evaluation. Finally the assessment framework should be relatable to a framework for treatment.

A clinical phonological assessment of child speech needs to consist of the following essential analytical procedures:

*Phonetic inventory*: states the phonetic characteristics of the child's pronunciation patterns.

*Contrastive assessments*: identify the phonetic and phonological matches and mismatches between the child and adult patterns; thereby assessing the communicative potential of the child's pronunciation patterns.

*Developmental assessment*: identifies the developmental status of the child's pronunciation patterns. (Grunwell, 1985)

For a well-founded treatment plan it is necessary for a full phonological assessment to be carried out based on a representative sample of the child's spontaneous speech.

The phonological evaluation of this assessment poses the following questions:

- Are the child's pronunciation patterns developmentally normal or not?
- If some patterns are normal, what is their developmental status relative to the child's age and *vis-à-vis* each other?
- If some patterns are not normal, are there identifiable sources of (or causes for) the emergence of developmentally abnormal patterns?
- In what ways are the child's pronunciation patterns different from the adult pronunciation patterns?
- Where there are differences, what are the implications for the child's ability to signal meaning differences?
- Are there any indications of phonological change; for example variability?
- Are the child's pronunciation patterns adequate to his/her communicative potential?

The answers given to these questions provide the information for planning the treatment programme. The framework for treatment derives from the same concepts as the framework for assessment. It is essential:

- to distinguish between phonetic and phonological treatment aims;
- to identify precisely the communicative inadequacies in the child's phonological patterns.

With regard to the latter, clinical research (Grunwell and Russell, 1990; 1991) has led to the identification of three parameters on which phonological patterns can be classified:

*Stability:* the consistency of the child's realisations of the adult tagets; or the amount of variability in these realisations.
*System*: the size of the child's phonetic inventory and contrastive system.
*Structure*: the distribution and combinations of consonants and the syllabic structures in the child's pronunciation patterns.

These three parameters form the focus of the decision-making principles.

### Remediation

Before delineating these principles a perspective on remediation will be developed. The purpose of speech therapy intervention is to bring about change in pronunciation patterns. For children with developmental speech disorders this is essentially assistance through a learning process which has apparently proved difficult for them. Learning to pronounce entails the maturation and mastery of oral motor skills, and the learning of the organisation and the establishment of cognitive knowledge of the sound system of the language.

As has already been indicated, children may need assistance in both aspects of this learning process. Examination of the process of both normal and disordered speech development suggests that there are two fundamental forces influencing the process: a tendency to establish rule-governed, or systematically patterned, speech production; a tendency to function initially with a simple speech sound system and gradually increase its complexity, building upon and extending existing abilities.

Remediation procedures should take advantage of these tendencies. As will be seen, the treatment principles outlined below do so. These two tendencies, and the remediation procedures, must operate within the constraints of the individual's speech sound-producing mechanism which determine output potential.

The creation of phonological knowledge may be affected by three types of constraints.

• Restricted perceptual encoding potential which may lead to a failure to store adequately less familiar phonetic elements; thus a child's information about the phonological characteristics of a word may be incomplete.

- Output constraints which limit a child's ability to produce certain articulatory targets or sequences; these may restrict a child's pronunciation patterns or result in avoidance of certain words.
- Organisational contraints which may operate on a child's output patterns in the production of certain targets; whereas in other types of targets the child demonstrates the required perceptual and articulatory abilities.

It has long been appreciated that each child presents with an individual profile and requires an individual programme. Approaches to facilitation should therefore be child centred, with strategies specifically designed to assist the child to overcome or compensate for particular constraints.

### Seven Decision-making Principles for Treatment Planning

1. Variability should be targeted in order to establish stable and accurate realisations.
2. The system of contrasts should be expanded to increase communicative adequacy.
3. New contrasts should be introduced first in well-established structures.
4. The phonotactic potential should be extended to increase communicative adequacy.
5. New structures should be introduced using well-established consonants.
6. Where possible the treatment programme should follow the normal developmental sequence.
7. Where appropriate the patterns that should be targeted first are those that are:
   (a) most deviant from the normal sequence of development;
   (b) most destructive of communicative adequacy in regard to the child's linguistic abilities.

As will be evident there are interrelationships between these seven principles: 1, 2 and 4 are the primary principles; 3 is a corollary to 2 as is 5 to 4; 6 and 7 are general guidelines to be applied when taking decisions relating to 1, 2 and 4 and when deciding the priorities between these three. Each of the principles will now be discussed and illustrated using longitudinal data of children receiving speech therapy.

### Variability

Variability is an important treatment target, not only because its eradication promotes communicative adequacy but also because it often indicates incipient change. An unstable system is, potentially, a changing system. (Grunwell, 1981). There are different types of variability and they have different implications for intervention.

Menn (1979) identified six types of variability in her investigation of normal phonological development. Clinical experience suggests that all six types occur in the speech of children with disordered development. The first type Menn calls *transitional variation;* this involves the gradual spread of a sound change across words involving the same target sound. Some words are pronounced only with the new form, others retain the old form and some are pronounced variably with the old and new form. This also known as *lexical diffusion.* Clearly this type of variability is potentially progressive and is an ideal treatment target for the establishment of a new contrast. The five other types of variability Menn regards as short term. In the clinical context, however, their implications warrant further investigation.

*Backgrounding* (or *trade-off;* Garnica and Edwards, 1977) involves regression in the pronunciation of one part of a word co-occurring with progress in another. It is important to be aware of this type of variability during treatment and to monitor its occurrence, bearing in mind that it is normally short term. *Imitation effect* occurs when a child's pronunciation of a word is very different when modelled. Most clinicians regard this as an indication of a child's potential ability; what must be remembered is that this does not necessarily imply easy incorporation into the child's habitual patterns. *Floundering* is the occurrence of wide fluctuation in the pronunciation of a word; this phenomenon suggests that the child has no stable concept of its sound structure. In the clinical context attention should be paid to where children flounder; it may indicate which sounds or sound sequences cause production difficulties and/or perceptual confusions or overload. *Lexical variation* is evident when certain words are highly variable while similar words are not. The implications for treatment planning of this phenomenon are not clear. The sixth and final type of variability is *rule coexistence* which is evidenced when children have two different forms of the same lexical item, or of the same target, that are not indicative of transitional variation. This occurs in the clinical context especially where there is extreme variability and a large number of instances of many-to-many correspondences between child and adult realisations. Treatment targets should attempt to disentangle this confusion. The illustration which follows exemplifies this.

Before presenting this illustration, a summary of types of variability that have the potential for developmental change follows.

*Progressive Phonological Variability*

1. Potential phonemic contrast

/t/ ⟶ [t]

/k/ ⟶ [k]

/k/ is realised correctly sometimes; if this became stable a new contrast would be established.

2. potential phonotactic extension (or derestriction), e.g. context conditioned variability such as context sensitive voicing where both voiced and voiceless sounds occur but in mutually exclusive contexts; if the occurrence of both is generalised to all contexts a new contrast would be established.

*Progressive Phonetic Variability*

1. Potential phonetic stability

/s/ ⟶ [s]

⟶ [ts]

correct /s/ realisations need to become stable

2. Potential phonetic maturation

/sl/  [ɸl]  ) context conditional
/sm/  [m̥ m]  ) variable phonetic
/sn/  [n̥ n]  ) correspondence

These /s/ realisations in clusters are a transition to the correct pronunciation of /s/; which process could be accelerated by intervention.

Neil provides an example of extreme variability (Grunwell and Russell, 1990). The Contrastive Assessment at 26/1 and 8/2 (Figure 17.1) reveals highly variable matches for most target phonemes across all positions. Analysis of these matches, using the PACS procedure for identifying Multiple Loss of Phonemic Contrasts (Figure 17.2) demonstrates the number of targets realised by several of Neil's consonant phones. It is evident that [d] and [g] are 'overworked' and are frequently used for the same targets. The first priority in the treatment plan for Neil was to reduce the variability. A word-based approach (see further below) was selected focusing on words with Syllable Initial Word Initial (SIWI) /t/ and /g/. These two target phonemes were chosen because in terms of their phonetic content they are the two phones used variably which are most different in feature content; they differ in both voicing and place.

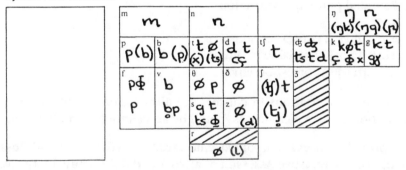

**Figure 17.1** Neil: Contrastive Assessment 26/1 and 8/2.

Furthermore there is an important functional difference in the way in which they are used: Neil's [g] realises a large number of targets SIWI, whereas Neil's [t] is seldom used for any other target except /t/ in this position. Because of the considerable overlapping it was not possible to select a pair of phones where the variability simply entailed a potential for change.

**Multiple Loss of Phonemic Contrasts**

| Child's Contrastive Phone | Target Phonemes Realized SIWI | Target Phonemes Realized SIWW | Target Phonemes Realized SFWF |
|---|---|---|---|
| p | p b | p | p (b) f θ |
| b | p b t v | b (p) v ð | b (p) v |
| t | t ʧ v s | s | t d ʧ ʤ k g s ʃ |
| d | t d ʤ k g f θ ð s z ʃ | t d θ z | d ʤ |
| k | k ʧ s | k t s ʃ | k g |
| g | t d ʧ k g f s (z) ʃ l | t d ʧ ʤ k g v ð s z ʃ ʒ h | s |
| w | w ɹ l | w t | |
| | | | |
| | | | |
| | | | |
| | | | |
| | | | |
| | | | |
| | | | |

**Feature Contrasts**

| | SIWI | SIWW | SFWF |
|---|---|---|---|
| Nasal − Plosive | | | |
| Stop − Fricative | | | |
| Stop − Affricate | | | |
| Fricative − Affricate | | | |
| Stop − Approximant | | | |
| Fricative − Approximant | | | |
| Labial − Lingual | | | |
| Alveolar − Velar | | | |
| Alveolar − Post-Alveolar | | | |
| Alveolar − Dental | | | |
| Voiced − Voiceless | | | |
| Med. Approx. − Lat. Approx. | | | |
| Other Features | | | |
| | | | |
| | | | |
| | | | |

**Figure 17.2** Neil: Multiple Loss of Phonemic Contrasts, 26/1 and 8/2.

Five months later, a second Contrastive Assessment at 18/7 and 19/7 (Figure 17.3) reveals that the realisations of all target plosive phonemes were stabilised and consistently correct across all word positions. The variability was now evident in the realisations of fricative targets (see further below). Notwithstanding, Neil was now intelligible, largely as a consequence of the eradication of the extreme variability.

**Syllable Initial Word Initial**

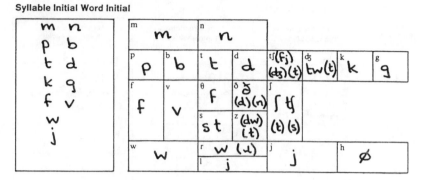

**Syllable Initial Within Word**

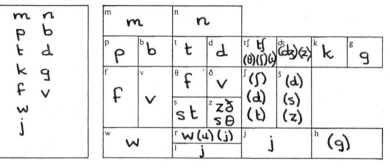

**Syllable Final Word Final**

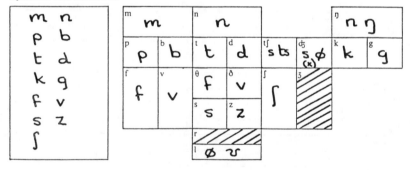

**Figure 17.3** Neil: Contrastive Assessment, 18/7 and 19/7.

## System Expansion

System expansion involves the introduction of new consonants that create new phonemic contrasts within the child's pronunciation patterns. The contrasts that are absent are revealed by the Phonetic Inventory and the Contrastive Assessment. In selecting the position(s) in which to introduce new contrasts, the guideline to target well-established structures first should be considered, though not necessarily rigidly applied (see further below). In introducing new consonant sounds phonetic factors often need to be addressed; these, however, are not the focus of this chapter and will therefore just be mentioned.

Neil once again provides an illustration of system expansion (Grunwell and Russell, 1990). The Phonetic Inventory 26/1 and 8/2 (Figure 17.4)

| | Labial | Dental | Alveolar | Post-Alveolar | Palatal | Velar | Glottal | Other |
|---|---|---|---|---|---|---|---|---|
| Nasal | m | | n | | | ŋ | | |
| Plosive | p b | | t d | | | k g | ʔ | |
| Fricative | ɸ | | | | ç | | h | |
| Affricate | | | | | | | | |
| Approximant | w | | l | | j | | | |
| Other | | | | | | | | |

Marginal Phones: ʃ ; f ; s ; x ; ʤ ; ɣ

## Phonetic Distribution

| | Single Consonants | | | | | Consonant Clusters | | | |
|---|---|---|---|---|---|---|---|---|---|
| | SIWI | SIWW | SFWW | SFWF | | SIWI | SIWW | SFWW | SFWF |
| Nasal | m n | m n | m n ŋ | m n ŋ | | bw pw gw gj | bw | | ŋts nt |
| Plosive | p b t d k g | p b t d k g ʔ | | p b t d k g | | | | | ɣ pɸ |
| Fricative | h | f¹ | s¹ | | | | | | ŋk |
| Affricate | | | | | | | | | |
| Approximant | w l j | w l j | | | | | | | |
| Other | | | | | | | | | |

**Figure 17.4** Neil: Phonetic Inventory, 26/1 and 8/2.

and Contrastive Assessment (Figure 17.1) reveal a major restriction in the types of consonants Neil used; fricatives and affricates are almost entirely lacking. With regard to Phonetic Distribution the inventory is well distributed across all four positions. While variability was the first priority, the lack of friction came a close second. In order to expand the potential to signal contrasts, new contrasts using the fricative feature needed to be established. It was decided to use a system-based approach (see further below) to introduce the /p/ – /f/ contrast through minimal pairs in SIWI position. This plosive-fricative contrast was chosen because they are phonetically distant from the other targets /t/ and /g/; SIWI position was chosen because it may be easier, given that Neil's inventory had balanced distribution. It was also noted that [f] is developmentally often the first fricative.

Five months later, the Phonetic Inventory 18/7 and 19/7 (Figure 17.5) demonstrates that fricatives had become established. Neil's realisations of the treatment target /f/ were stable, see Contrastive Assessment 18/7 and 19/7 (Figure 17.3). Furthermore, lingual fricatives had developed but were not yet fully established. It is noteworthy that the position in which they were most stable is Syllable Final Word Final (SFWF); Ferguson (1978) suggests that fricatives often develop first in SFWF. Not only had Neil spontaneously generalised the new fricative feature, the voiced/voiceless contrast had become established for plosives and fricatives. This, it can be assumed, is a consequence of the judicious selection of the voiceless plosive and fricative contrast in SIWI where the realisations were voiced. This is an example of where a contrast is not directly targeted, but indirectly introduced through considered choice of other targets. While not having the status of a treatment principle, the consideration of the overall phonetic configuration of the child's system is an important factor in treatment strategies.

## Structural Expansion; Extension of Phonotactic Potential and Introduction of New Structures

Structural expansion involves the introduction of new phonotactic patterns that create new contrastive phonological units within the child's pronunciation patterns. The Phonetic Inventory and Contrastive Assessments often reveal maldistribution of consonant phones. In seeking to establish new distributional patterns, the guideline to use well established consonants should be given first consideration, though not necessarily rigidly adhered to (see further below).

Helen provides an illustration of structural expansion (Grunwell and Russell, 1991). The Contrastive Assessment at 10/88 (Figure 17.6) reveals that the major restriction in Helen's pronunciation patterns is in regard to distributional possibilities: there is a complete absence of SFWF consonants. There are, furthermore, severe phonotactic constraints on word structure. Of 50 disyllables in the sample, 20 are reduced to mono-syllables and five out of eight polysyllabic words are reduced. These phonotactic restrictions were the first treatment targets using rhythm exer-cises and then the production of reduplicated and nonreduplicated CVCV words containing the well-established plosive and nasal consonants.

| | Labial | Dental | Alveolar | Post-Alveolar | Palatal | Velar | Glottal | Other |
|---|---|---|---|---|---|---|---|---|
| Nasal | m | | n | | | ŋ | | |
| Plosive | p b | | t d | | | k g | | |
| Fricative | f v | θ ð | s z | ʃ | | | | |
| Affricate | | | | ʧ ʤ | | | | |
| Approximant | w | | | ɹ | j | | | |
| Other | | | | | | | | |

Marginal Phones:  ʔ x

## Phonetic Distribution

| | Single Consonants | | | | | Consonant Clusters | | | |
|---|---|---|---|---|---|---|---|---|---|
| | SIWI | SIWW | SFWW | SFWF | | SIWI | SIWW | SFWW | SFWF |
| Nasal | m n | m n | m n ŋ | m n ŋ | | pj bw bj | pj bw | | mp nt nd |
| Plosive | p b t d k g | p b t d k g | p t k | p b t d k g | | tw tɹ dw kw | tw | | nʤ ns nz |
| Fricative | f v θ ð s ʃ | f v θ s z ʃ | f θ s | f v s z ʃ | | kj qw gj | gw | | ɸs ts ks |
| Affricate | ʧ | ʧ ʤ | | | | fj | fj | | |
| Approximant | w ɹ j | w j | | | | m̥m n̥n | | | |
| Other | | | | | | | | | |

**Figure 17.5** Neil: Phonetic Inventory, 18/7 and 19/7.

The second target was SFWF position in monosyllabic CVC words; once again nasals were selected.

Five months later (Figure 17.7) it is evident from the Contrastive Assessment (Helen 3/89) that SFWF consonants are now well established, in particular nasals, voiceless plosives and voiced fricatives. There is variability, especially in the realisations of the spontaneously introduced sibilants both in Word Final and Within Word Positions. With regard to the phonotactic structure of words, of 56 disyllabic words only three are reduced and out of eight polysyllabic words, three are reduced.

**Syllable Initial Word Initial**

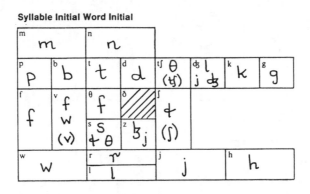

**Syllable Initial Within Word**

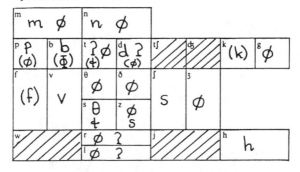

**Syllable Final Word Final**

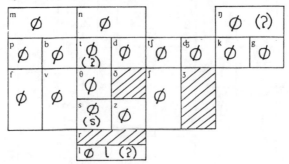

**Figure 17.6** Helen: Contrastive Assessment, 10/88.

It is clear that Helen had overcome the phonotactic constraints evidenced in the previous assessment.

It is interesting to reflect upon the spontaneous development of a wide range of SFWF consonants when only nasals were targeted. This pattern of change has been noted in two other cases (Grunwell and Russell, 1991) where the treatment strategy of introducing reduplicated and non-reduplicated disyllabic CVCV words was used. In Helen's case these structures were targeted in order to establish disyllabic words. In retrospect, however, perhaps this target might also have promoted and supported

**Syllable Initial Word Initial**

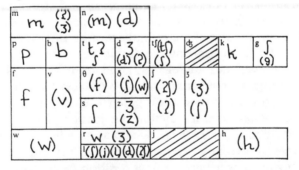

**Syllable Initial Within Word**

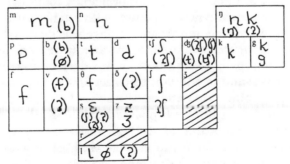

**Syllable Final Word Final**

**Figure 17.7** Helen: Contrastive Assessment, 3/89.

the development of SFWF consonants. In normal development, reduplication has been found to be an early pattern co-occurring with Final Consonant Deletion and preceding the emergence of final consonants. The occurrence and functions of reduplication are controversial (Fee and Ingram, 1982; Ferguson, 1983; Grunwell, 1987; Ingram, 1989; Lahey, Flax and Schlisselberg, 1985; Schwartz et al., 1980). One of the functions identified explicitly by Ferguson (1983) is that 'it is a means to facilitate the use of syllable-closing consonants'. This would account for the spontaneous generalisation observed in Helen's pronunciation patterns.

*Developmental Sequence*

The developmental sequence has been frequently advanced as a guiding principle in treatment planning (Jakobson, 1968; Ingram, 1989; Hodson and Paden, 1991). There appear to be two reasons adduced for its justification: it provides a measure of complexity in that those patterns that occur earlier in the developmental sequence are taken to be easier; it represents a return to normality in that disordered phonological development entails some deviation(s) from the normal sequence, such that treatment targets that reflect that sequence rectify the deviation(s). As indicated above, reference to the developmental sequence can be invoked as a guiding principle for any treatment decision indeed, in the above illustrations for both system expansion and structural expansion developmental factors were referred to in the selection of the fricative to target for Neil and the use of the reduplication strategy for Helen.

A further example of applying the developmental principle is the case of Andrew (Grunwell and Russell, 1991). At 10/88 (Figure 17.8) Andrew used a small range of consonant sounds; notably he has no oral fricatives. In addition his pronunciation patterns show major distributional restrictions; Final Consonant Deletion is evidenced for all obstruent targets. It was decided to target these two areas of deficiency simultaneously by one strategy, evoking the developmental principle that fricatives have been shown to occur first in final position (Ferguson, 1978). It was recognised that this ran counter to the principles about new contrasts in established structures and new structures with established sounds.

Seven months later no appreciable change was detected in Andrew's patterns. There appeared a number of extraneous reasons for this. However, the treatment plan was reviewed; it was decided to continue to target SFWF fricatives and in addition to target SIWW consonants to eradicate the deviant glottal stop pattern. The second aim was targeted using reduplicated and then non-reduplicated CVCV words containing the well established plosives and nasals. Four months later at 9/89 (Figure 17.9) it is evident that some fricatives were established at SFWF position and spontaneously generalised to other positions; indeed all types of consonants were now present SFWF (cf. Helen above).

## *Targeting Patterns*

The principle that *deviant and destructive patterns* should be targeted first relates to all six preceding principles. Clinical experience suggests that the most deviant patterns often are, or are part of, the destructive patterns.

Marcus provides an illustration of a child with a very deviant pronunciation pattern (Grunwell and Russell, 1991). In 5/89 Marcus' range of consonants was [n (b) t d k g n l (w)] (Figure 17.10). These were only

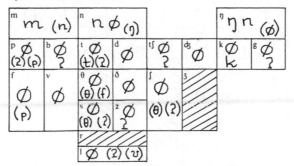

**Figure 17.8** Andrew: Contrastive Assessment, 10/88.

used in SIWI position. There is complete absence of SFWF consonants; in SIWW position it was unrealistic to attempt a Contrastive Assessment because of the prevalence of Assimilation patterns i.e. Consonant Harmony, Reduplication and Metathesis. These patterns also account for the extreme variability in SIWI position. The occurrence of [b] as a realisation of SIWI /m/ and of [n̥ᶠc] for /s; ʃ/ is an extremely unusual phenomenon.

The first aim of treatment was to strengthen the weakest consonants in SIWI position which were [m p b w]. This also entailed targeting one

**Syllable Initial Word Initial**

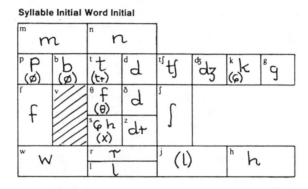

**Syllable Initial Within Word**

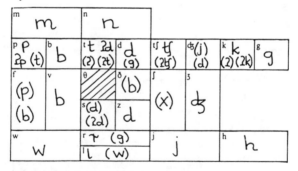

**Syllable Final Word Final**

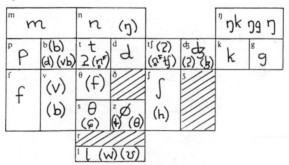

**Figure 17.9** Andrew: Contrastive Assessment, 9/89.

of the most deviant aspects of his patterns in that these labial consonants
are normally established first. The second aim was introduced after 10
weeks' intensive therapy; this was to improve the limited and unusual
phonotactic patterns. The strategy applied was the production of non-
reduplicated CVCV words using established SIWI nasal and plosives.
Non-reduplicated words only were used to break down the assimilation
patterns. By 2/90 (Figure 17.11) changes consistent with the treatment
strategy were evident. In addition, spontaneous development of SFWF
consonants was evident (cf. Helen and Andrew above; Grunwell and

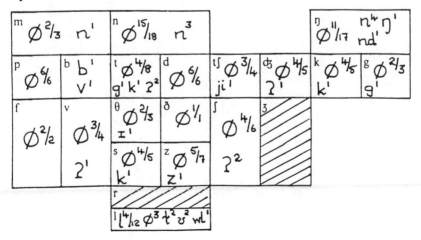

Figure 17.10 Marcus: Contrastive Assessment, 5/89.

Russell; 1991). There are clearly many more changes that needed to be facilitated in Marcus' pronunciation patterns; nonetheless positive and appreciable progress was occurring. As with most very unusual pronunciation patterns treatment is long term, and the programme is evolving and to an extent experimental; the changing patterns should be monitored frequently and closely so that treatment aims and strategies are responsive to the child's needs.

## Syllable Initial Word Initial

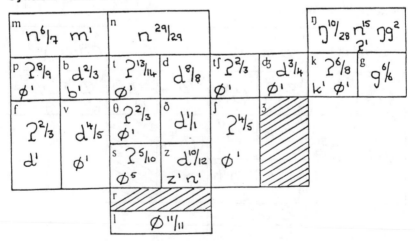

## Syllable Final Word Final

**Figure 17.11** Marcus: Contrastive Assessment, 2/90.

## Treatment Strategies

As is evident from the above discussion the seven decision-making principles enable the clinician to identify treatment targets in an explicitly principled way. The philosophy upon which these principles are based also engenders particular approaches to treatment itself. The focus is on patterns of pronunciation rather than on individual sounds. The treatment materials highlight the functions of pronunciation patterns, that is to transmit meaning and signal meaningful contrasts. The primary strategy in treatment, therefore, is to control the child's linguistic environment such that it promotes and facilitates the phonological changes that have been identified as treatment targets (Gibbon and Grunwell, 1990). The theoretical assumption underlying this strategy is that phonological development is sensitive to input (Ingram, 1986). There are two types of techniques that a clinician may use in applying this strategy : these could be called meta-linguistic and manipulative. Meta-linguistic techniques involve what has been called above a system-based approach; the child is deliberately exposed to examples of the phonological system 'at work'. This occurs for example during auditory discrimination exercises involving minimal pairs, minimal pair contrast therapy in production exercises, homonymy/homophony confrontation and exercises to develop meta-linguistic awareness such as the Metaphon approach (Dean et al.,1990). Manipulative techniques involve what has been called above a word-based approach; the child is exposed to a considerably increased number of examples of a selected target type of phonological unit. This occurs for example when the listening technique of 'auditory bombardment' is used (Hodson and Paden, 1991); when word lists are drawn up for the child to practise certain types of sounds or structures and when sentences and stories are constructed for, and often by, the child, containing words exemplifying particular sounds and structures (i.e. 'phonologically loaded narratives'). The last technique frequently involves a combination of both the manipulative and the metalinguistic, since minimal pairs are sometimes incorporated into the names of people and objects featured in the story.

Another aspect of controlling the environment is the selection of the phonological and phonetic contexts in which the targets are presented. Principles 3 and 5 deal with this to some extent. There are other dimensions of the context that may need to be controlled such as the other consonants in the syllable or word; the length of the word, phrase or clause; the vowels preceding or following a target consonant. To illustrate the last factor as an example of the point at issue, alveolar plosives [t d] are apparently easier before front vowels and velar plosives [k g] easier before back vowels; this is phonetically logical; it could usefully be employed as a facilitating strategy for a child with problems producing one or both types of consonants.

The aim of this section has been to emphasise that clinicians need to be explicit not only in identifying and justifying treatment aims but also in selecting and explaining their treatment strategies and techniques.

## Processes of Phonological Change

As indicated at the beginning of this chapter treatment planning is not just the devising of a programme on the basis of an initial assessment, it includes the monitoring and modification of the programme as the child's pronunciation patterns begin to change. Clinical experience suggests that there are four basic types or processes of phonological change:

stabilisation;
destabilisation;
innovation;
generalisation.

*Stabilisation* involves the resolution of a variable pronunciation pattern into a stable pattern. *Destabilisation* involves the disruption of a stable pattern resulting in variability. *Innovation* involves the introduction of a new pattern. *Generalisation* involves the transfer of a pronunciation pattern from one context to another. Generalisation as a process of change is a traditional focus in clinical practice; Appendix 1 summarises the different types of generalisation that are sought (cf. Gibbon and Grunwell, 1990). The focus here is on the processes themselves, their functions and interrelationships. Stabilisation occurs where there is variability an unstable or destabilised pattern; stabilisation leads to predictable relationships and potential progressive change through the establishment of new contrasts. Destabilisation occurs where there is stability; destabilisation may be caused by innovation or generalisation. Destabilisation may lead to potential progressive change if the resultant variability is ultimately resolved by stabilisation. Innovation occurs when a new pattern appears or is introduced; this may initially result in destabilisation of existing patterns and the creation of variability eventually leading to stabilisation of the new pattern and progressive change. Innovation may also lead to generalisation. Generalisation of one pattern to a new context as indicated previously may initially result in destabilisation of the existing pattern and variability, ultimately leading to stabilisation of the new pattern.

Awareness of these processes, their interrelationships and outcomes is useful in monitoring change and modifying treatment aims in an ongoing treatment programme. A final illustration demonstrates this point and the application of the principles and guidelines discussed in this paper. Marcus by 9/90 (Figure 17.12) had achieved much more regular pronunciation patterns than at the beginning of the year. Having regard to his stage of development, the next contrast to be established should involve a lingual fricative. The variable realisations of /ʃ/ - [f] suggest that this may be a point of potential change and that /ʃ/ might be a target susceptible to innovation. Manipulative word-based strategies were employed targeting /ʃ/ in all three word positions and carefully controlling contexts to involve well established nasals and plosives, avoiding [g] as this is a variable realisation of /ʃ/. When these exercises were established, a different set of techniques involving auditory

**Syllable Initial Word Initial**

**Syllable Initial Within Word**

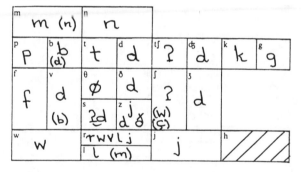

**Syllable Final Word Final**

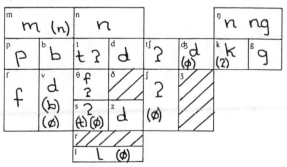

**Figure 17.12** Marcus: Contrastive Assessment, 9/90.

discrimination of fricatives in general and some production exercises were employed in an attempt to stimulate generalisation to all fricatives.

By 3/91 (Figure 17.13) appreciable changes can be detected. The introduction of /ʃ/ has been successful and there has been generalisation to affricates /tʃ/ and /dʒ/, most successfully in SIWI position, which is predictable since the previous realisations were Velars, the same as /ʃ/. The realisations of affricates in SIWW and SFWF have been destabilised by innovation through partial generalisation. These patterns need to be fully generalised and stabilised.

**Syllable Initial Word Initial**

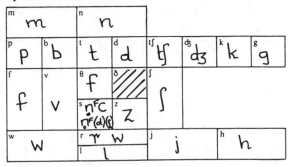

**Syllable Initial Within Word**

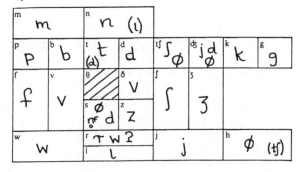

**Syllable Final Word Final**

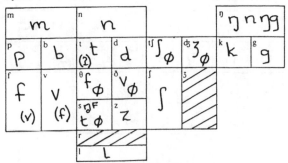

**Figure 17.13** Marcus: Contrastive Assessment, 3/91.

The other fricative realisations have also undergone change with the introduction of /v/ in all contexts and its generalisation to / ð /, a developmentally normal realisation; /z/ is also present in all positions. The next target is clearly /s/ which will involve innovation. It might be anticipated that this will prove a resistant target as the realisations in SIWI are very unusual involving a sound not known to occur in natural languages and patterns of addition, Consonant Harmony and Metathesis; all factors that Leonard (1985) has identified as indicators of unusual phonological behaviour. These factors lead to a decision to target /s/ first in SFWF position, in which position it often first emerges in normal development.

## Conclusion

The aim of this chapter has been to discuss issues which influence decision making in treatment planning. It has delineated and illustrated principles that will enable clinicians to make explicit and formalise the decision-making process. A firmer foundation for predicting outcome is thus created. The importance of monitoring and responding to emergent developments has been emphasised. A framework in which such phonological changes can be identified, evaluated and managed has been suggested. By applying this framework clinicians are able to make principled decisions in ongoing treatment planning.

## References

DEAN, E, HOWELL, J., HILL, A. and WALTERS, D. (1990). *Metaphon Resource Pack.* Windsor: NFER–Nelson.

FEE, J. and INGRAM, D. (1982). Reduplication as a strategy of phonological development. *Journal of Child Language,* 9, 41–54.

FERGUSON, C.A. (1978). Fricatives in child language acquisition. In: Honsa, V. and Hardman-de-Bautista, M.J. (Eds), *Papers on Linguistics and Child Language: Ruth Hirsh Weir Memorial Volume.* The Hague: Mouton.

FERGUSON, C.A. (1983). Reduplication in child phonology. *Journal of Child Language,* 10, 239–243.

GARNICA, O. and EDWARDS, M. (1977). Phonological variation in child speech – the trade-off phenomenon. *Ohio State University Working Papers in Linguistics,* 22, 81–87.

GIBBON, F. and GRUNWELL, P. (1990). Specific developmental language learning difficulties. In: Grunwell, P. (Ed.), *Developmental Speech Disorders.* Edinburgh: Churchill Livingstone.

GRUNWELL, P. (1981). *The Nature of Phonological Disability in Children.* London: Academic Press.

GRUNWELL, P. (1985). *Phonological Assessment of Child Speech.* (PACS). Windsor: NFER-Nelson.

GRUNWELL, P. (1987). *Clinical Phonology,* 2nd edn. London: Croom Helm.

GRUNWELL, P. (1988). Phonological assessment, evaluation and explanation of speech disorders in children. *Clinical Linguistics and Phonetics,* 2, 221–252.

GRUNWELL, P. (1989). Developmental phonological disorders and normal speech development: a review and illustration. *Child Language Teaching and Therapy*, 5, 304–319.

GRUNWELL, P. (Ed.) (1990). *Developmental Speech Disorders*. Edinburgh: Churchill Livingstone.

GRUNWELL, P. and RUSSELL, J. (1990). A phonological disorder in an English-speaking child: a case study. *Clinical Linguistics and Phonetics*, 4, 29–38.

GRUNWELL, P. and RUSSELL, J. (1991). Patterns of change in phonological disorders. Paper presented at Second Conference of European Child Language Disorders Research Group, Roros, 1990. To be published in the Proceedings by The Norwegian Centre for Child Research.

HODSON, B.W. and PADEN, E.P. (1991). *Targeting Intelligible Speech*, 2nd edn. Austin, TX: Pro-Ed.

INGRAM, D. (1986). Explanation and phonological remediation. *Child Language Teaching and Therapy*, 2, 1–16.

INGRAM, D. (1989). *Phonological Disability in Children*, 2nd edn. London: Whurr.

JAKOBSON, R. (1968). *Child Language, Aphasia and Phonological Universals*. The Hague: Mouton.

LAHEY, M. FLAX,. J. and SCHLISSELBERG, G. (1985). A preliminary investigation of reduplication in children with specific language impairment. *Journal of Speech and Hearing Disorders*, 50, 186–194.

LANCASTER, G. and POPE, L. (1989). *Working with Children's Phonology*. Bicester: Winslow Press.

LEONARD, L.D. (1985). Unusual and subtle phonological behavior in the speech of phonologically disordered children. *Journal of Speech and Hearing Disorders*, 50, 4–13.

MENN, L. (1979) Transition and variation in child phonology. Modelling a developing system. In *Proceedings of the 9th International Congress of Phonetic Sciences, Copenhagen.* Vol. II.

SCHWARTZ, R.G., LEONARD, L.D., WILCOX, M.J. and FOLGER, M.K. (1980). Again and again: reduplication in child phonology. *Journal of Child Language*, 7, 75–87.

SHRIBERG, L.D., KWIATKOWSKI, J., BEST, S., HENGST, J. and TERSELIC-WEBER, B. (1986). Characteristics of children with phonologic disorders of unknown origin. *Journal of Speech and Hearing Disorders*, 51, 140–161.

## Appendix 17.1 Types of generalisation in phonological change

Transfer of phonological skills may occur across four contexts:
*Phonological*
• From one syllabic position to another
• From one target phoneme to another (usually in the same sound class)
*Lexical*
• from one word to all the others in which the target phoneme occurs
*Syntactic*
• From one type of linguistic unit (e.g. single word) to larger linguistic units (phrases, clauses, conversation)
*Socioenvironmental*
• From the clinic to all environments and all types of discourse

# Chapter 18
# Early screening and intervention

DAVID M.B. HALL

The term 'Screening' is often applied to any kind of active case-finding process, but the concept actually refers to:

> the use of simple tests or procedures to check persons who believe themselves to be healthy, in order to detect some abnormality or disease process which is not yet clinically obvious and whose prognosis will be improved by early treatment.

This chapter should perhaps be entitled 'Early *detection* and intervention', since screening is only one aspect of early detection. I shall consider what methods of early detection are available for problems of speech and language development; what precisely we are hoping to detect; the advantages and disadvantages of screening; and finally the alternative strategies available to us.

## Terminology

On both sides of the Atlantic there has been continuing debate among paediatricians and epidemiologists about terminology in relation to developmental screening and surveillance, but a consensus is now emerging (Butler, 1989; Hall, Hill and Elliman ,1990). The term 'Health Promotion' describes a philosophical approach; it is 'the process of enabling people to take control of, and accept responsibility for, their own health'.

Within this concept, there are three areas of professional activity: health education, health protection and disease prevention. These concepts overlap; for example, health education plays an important role in disease prevention. Health education involves the provision of information and advice in a way that is acceptable to the individual or to the community and is intended to bring about some enduring change in health related behaviour. All of us are involved in this to a greater or lesser extent. Health protection is mainly to do with environmental regulation, for example the design of road layouts or playgrounds to avoid accidents, the provision of suitable day care that can facilitate rather than retard a child's development – or the banning of pit bull terriers.

Disease prevention is in turn subdivided into primary, secondary and tertiary prevention. Primary prevention refers to activities such as immunisation, which prevent a condition from happening in the first place. Secondary prevention is to do with reducing the prevalence of a condition by early detection and intervention. The term 'Child Health Surveillance' is used to describe all activities under this heading. Tertiary prevention refers to the reduction of the impact of an illness or disability on the child's life.

**Passive versus Active Detection**

When we as health professionals focus our attention on a particular problem which engages our interest, we can discern an evolution or progression in approach which seems to be repeated in a wide variety of conditions. I will illustrate my point by reference to malignant melanoma. Everyone has heard of this black pigmented skin tumour, which can be very malignant and deadly; and most people have probably looked anxiously at a mole on their person at some point in their lives!

The first stage in this progression was the identification of the condition, and its natural history was then documented. The predisposing factors, such as light skin colouring and excessive sun exposure, were established. It gradually became clear that early diagnosis and treatment would greatly improve the patient's chance of survival. In recent years, interest in the tumour increased because it seemed to become very much more common. It no longer seemed acceptable simply to wait for patients to present themselves at the specialist clinic for treatment. A more active approach was justifiable and several ideas were considered.

First, health education regarding the dangers of sunburn for those with light skin colour seemed desirable; this would pursue the aim of Primary Prevention. Secondly, since primary prevention would never totally eliminate the condition, early detection was required; in other words, Secondary Prevention. Since these tumours might appear at any time in a person's life, it was clearly not practicable to offer a screening programme. Instead, health education about the warning signs of malignancy was introduced; health professionals were taught what action should be undertaken; and access to special clinics for these patients was made rapid and simple.

There are a number of important ethical and practical considerations involved in the shift from the passive system to the active case-finding approach. In traditional practice, the unspoken contract between patient and professional is that the latter will do their best, within the skills and resources available, to diagnose, explain and solve the problem as presented to them. With active case finding (however it is undertaken) the contract is very different. The professionals are actually proclaiming

> You, the patient (or parent) may have some health problem, which you have not yet identified or have failed to acknowledge; but we have tests which will detect it; we can tell you whether any problem we find is significant; we can tell you if it needs treatment; we know that early treatment will improve the prognosis; and we can provide that treatment.

As professionals, we need to consider whether all these statements are true. Unless we are confident that we can deliver these promises, it is arguably unethical to initiate such active case finding.

## Impairments

The evolution of professional interest in specific language impairment (SLI) has followed a path similar to the one outlined for malignant melanoma. In clinical practice, ever since paediatrics was established as a speciality, parents have consulted their doctor or speech therapist, complaining that in their view (or the opinion of a friend or relative, or a playgroup leader) the child's language acquisition was delayed. Of course, no one doubts that parents should receive the best advice available.

The question to be addressed in this chapter is this: are we justified in undertaking active case finding for children who have delayed speech and language acquisition? In attempting to answer this question I shall consider the methods of case finding which are currently in use; examine the aims of this activity; and finally offer some practical proposals.

### Models of Active Detection

The literature suggests several models of how active detection might work. The first, and the easiest to deal with, is the developmental screening test. This is associated inevitably with the name of Frankenburg, who devised and researched the Denver Developmental Screening Test (DDST). Many other developmental screening tests have since been designed and used; some cover all areas of development, while others focus more specifically on speech and language. Since the DDST and

---

**(a)**

i) The condition being sought should be an important health problem for the individual and for the community.

ii) There should be an acceptable form of treatment for patients with recognisable disease or some other form of useful intervention should be available (e. g. genetic advice).

iii) The natural history of the condition, including its development from latent to declared disease, should be adequately understood.

iv) There should be a recognisable latent or early symptomatic stage.

v) There should be a suitable test or examination for detecting the disease at an early or latent stage, which should be acceptable to the population.

vi) Facilities should be available for diagnosing and treating the patients uncovered by this programme.

vii) There should be an agreed policy on whom to treat as patients.

viii) The treatment at the pre-symptomatic stage of the disease should favorably influence its course and prognosis.

ix) The cost of case finding which should include cost of diagnosis and treatment should be economically balanced in relation to (1) possible expenditure on medical care as a whole and (2) the cost of treatment if the patient does not present until the disease reaches the symptomatic stage.

x) Case finding should be a continuing process, not a once and for all project.

**(b) THE IDEAL SCREENING TEST IS:**

i) Simple, quick and easy to interpret: capable of being performed by paramedical or other personnel.

ii) Acceptable to the public, since participation in screening programmes is voluntary.

iii) Accurate, i.e. give a true measurement of the attribute under investigation.

iv) Repeatable. This involves the components of observer variability, both within and between tests; subject variability; test variability.

v) Sensitive. This is the ability of a test to give a positive finding when the individual screened has the disease or abnormality under investigation.

vi) Specific. This is the ability of the test to give a negative finding when the individual does not have the disease or abnormality under investigation.

**Figure 18.1** (a) The Wilson and Jungner criteria for a screening programme. (b) The Cochrane and Holland criteria for an ideal screening test.

many other similar tests have been widely used in North America, I shall for convenience call this the North American screening model.

The characteristic of the North American model is that the tests used fulfil, or are intended to fulfil, the well-known classic criteria for a screening procedure (Figure 18.1). Note in particular that screening tests should be simple and capable of use by paramedical staff and that there should be clear definition of what is meant by a case. The term 'screening' should not be used to describe a particular activity unless there is an intention to fulfil these criteria (see Hall, 1991).In the UK, the approach has been rather different. Children have been subjected to regular developmental examinations, but until recently these were usually carried out by doctors rather than paramedical staff; the procedures had no inbuilt pass–fail criteria and doctors were expected to use their judgment and common sense in deciding whether to refer the child for in-depth assessment. Although these examinations shared the objectives of screening, in that the aim was to examine a population of apparently normal children, it was clear that the procedure itself was not a screening test. Some authorities have nevertheless retained the term 'screening' for such examinations (Drillien and Drummond, 1983), while others have called this activity 'developmental surveillance'. I propose that for our purposes we call this the UK model of developmental screening.

Developmental examinations can be used as an opportunity for counselling parents on a variety of issues related to child health, growth and development. In the North American literature this is called developmental guidance. Some screening procedures make use of parental observations and require the parents to complete various checklists or questionnaires, but relatively little has been written on the role of health education or professional training as an adjunct to early detection, and even less on the subject of primary prevention.

## What is the Target Condition?

If we initiate an active case-finding programme for children with speech and language problems, what exactly are we to look for? Some authorities would regard 'delay in speech and language acquisition' as the target problem, whereas others would focus on SLI. Many would argue that a central role of any community developmental screening and surveillance programme is to discover children with language delay associated with deprivation, neglect and abuse.

Several factors may be associated with language delay and these might provide a basis for dividing children with language delay into subgroups. This might enable us to focus our early detection efforts on the children whose progress is most amenable to intervention. The five factors to be considered here are hearing loss, global learning difficulties, specific language impairment, autism and social deprivation.

### Children with Hearing Loss

The majority of children with sensorineural hearing loss should be detected before the age of three, but secretory otitis media (SOM) is very common and is believed by many to be an important contributory factor to language delay (Haggard and Hughes, 1991). The literature on this topic is vast but it can be summarised as follows:

- there is an association between SOM in early childhood and developmental delays, particularly in language;
- the association is not necessarily causal and is of small magnitude; both the severity and duration of the hearing loss and the vulnerability of the child probably affect the impact on development;
- SOM is common, but only a small minority of children have severe persistent disease. In most it is transient and self-limiting.

Although some authorities believe that we should screen all 3 year olds for SOM, there is as yet no evidence that such screening would be either practical or beneficial. It is probably more relevant to exclude SOM routinely at any age as a possible cause of language, learning or behavioural problems than to undertake universal screening for the condition itself.

### Children with Learning Difficulties

Three studies on the prognosis of language delay at 3 years indicate that a substantial proportion of these children have a full-scale IQ well below the mean (Silva, 1987); in other words, the presenting feature, slow language development, is the marker for other less obvious but more global learning difficulties. Much of the predictive value of slow language development for later school problems can be attributed to the global learning difficulty rather than to the delay in talking. The distribution of intelligence is of course continuous, so that no absolute distinction can be made between normal and slow-learning children.

### Children with SLI of Different Types

This is the group of particular interest to the present readership, although of course SLI children constitute a minority of those detected by a language screening programme. SLI children are a heterogeneous group. Phonological problems (which often worry parents a great deal) usually have a good prognosis in terms of overall language competence and educational progress. The children most likely to have persisting problems are those who have difficulty in conveying the theme of a simple story; in other words, who have a more wide-ranging difficulty in the use of language for communication (Bishop and Adams, 1990). The question of whether SLI is indeed an entity at all is still contentious. It now seems clear that the distinction between 'delay' and 'disorder' is not helpful in practice, hence the value of the term SLI which bypasses the need to make such distinctions. But does SLI represent a condition, or is it an artificial construct?

Leonard (1987) has argued that none of the hypothetical substrates of

SLI permit us to make an absolute distinction between SLI and 'normal' children. He suggests that we should not seek a specific cause for SLI because the problems of these children are:

> simply the product of the same types of variations in genetic and environmental factors that lead some children to be clumsy, others to be non-musical and still others to have little insight into feelings

The feature which seems most often to prompt professional concern is a discrepancy between different fields of development. This may apply either to lack of synchrony between various aspects of language acquisition, or to differences between, for example, verbal and non-verbal skills. But there is no reason to suppose that all individuals should show similar levels of ability in all aspects of mental functioning; we would expect discrepancies to show a distribution curve just like any other biological measurement.

If this reasoning is correct, it would follow that there can never be an absolute definition of SLI (or of autism or global learning difficulties) and therefore no watertight screening test. Elsewhere I have argued along similar lines in the case of clumsiness (developmental coordination disorder) and this view helps to make sense of the spectrum of autistic disorder (see below). The concept of a spectrum of impairment is more compatible with clinical observation than that of an entity which is either present or absent.

## Autistic Children

Many of the children who present with language delay or more global communication difficulties are also socially 'odd' and are often described as 'having autistic tendencies' or 'being a bit autistic', although everyone agrees that they are not classically autistic. Most authorities now believe that the key deficit in autism is social impairment and that social ability forms a continuum as does language ability (Wing, 1988; Bishop, 1989). The dimension of social competence and impairment adds further confusion to the question of screening. Often it is these socially impaired children who cause the most concern over the first few years of school and they are more difficult to help than those who are socially well integrated and responsive to adult and peer attention. Any screening method which concentrates on vocabulary and syntax, and fails to take account of the child's social skills and ability to communicate effectively, will miss a significant proportion of the potential problem children.

## *Social deprivation and language impairment*

Impairment of language acquisition is a common, though by no means invariable, feature of social deprivation and child abuse and neglect. Deprivation *can* be associated with both global developmental retardation and more specific impairment of language and social abilities. To some extent, however, the distinction between children who are slow to talk because of deprivation and those who are slow for some presumably more 'biological' or intrinsic reason, is artificial. Children who tend to be uncommunicative probably receive less input for that reason; and this is true whether the child is growing up in severely deprived circumstances or in a linguistically supportive environment.

### Labels or Profiles?

Although we can describe global intellectual deficits or specific language impairments as *causes* of delayed language acquisition, they are not really causes at all; they are simply ways of relabelling the observed phenomena. The dangers of labelling children have become increasingly obvious to clinicians and parents over the past decade, yet the need to label some children as having a developmental problem, and others as normal, is implicit in any screening procedure.

In our own clinical practice, we try to avoid the pitfalls of labelling by explaining to parents how each of the many dimensions of human development can vary along a continuous spectrum. The relationships

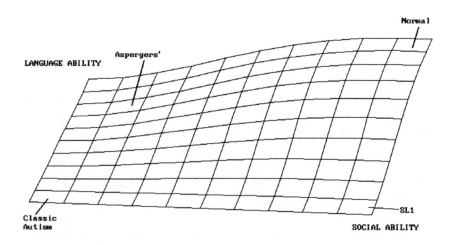

**Figure18.2** Three-dimensional graph to show relationship between language and social skills.

between social competence and language development are illustrated in Figure 18.2. We could equally well relate motor competence and language, or constructional competence and social skills. We would then find in the corners of the chart children with the 'clumsy child syndrome' or 'non-verbal learning disabilities'. This approach has increased the relevance of diagnostic evaluation; but it has made us realise how difficult it is to undertake screening for such problems.

## Problems of Screening for Language Delay

There are no simple ways of screening for global intellectual deficits, SLI, autistic behaviour patterns, or social deprivation. If screening is to be undertaken, the target phenomenon must surely be language delay itself, rather than any subgroup of 'delayed' children. All the possible causes and associations of language delay are potentially serious, but before we could devise a logical programme we would need to decide which aspects of language and what level of delay are to be selected in designing the screening procedures, and also at what age or ages screening should be undertaken. When we try to do this, a number of serious problems emerge, and these will now be reviewed in detail.

### The Definition of 'Delay'

The first and most obvious problem is to define 'delay'. Both the rate and the route of language acquisition vary widely within apparently normal children. For example, the distribution curves for Reynell Expressive language scores (Figure 18.3) illustrate how a child aged 4 years may be advanced or delayed by 18 months or more and yet be within two standard deviations of the mean (Wells, 1985). In order to appreciate the difficulties of interpreting the significance of a 'low' language score, it may be helpful to consider another medical analogy, that of height.

The Reynell curves might equally well represent the heights of children. If a child's height falls near the − 2 s.d. line, we do not say that he is 'growth delayed'. We simply regard him as a short child. We expect that he may have small parents and that he may well turn out not to be very tall as an adult. Unfortunately, measurements alone do not help us to discover which children have a treatable condition, like hormonal deficiency, and which are just normal short children. Even children whose height is below the third centile are probably normal; conversely, a child whose height is well above the third centile may still have a growth disorder. The best way to discover growth disorders is to take serial measures, but even with such a simple parameter as height, this turns out to be very difficult.

Similar considerations apply to language development. Some of the children who fail a language screening test may be deaf, or mentally handicapped, or autistic, or suffering severe deprivation; but these problems may also be found in children whose language is sufficient for them to pass a screening test. In the literature on language screening, authors vary in their choice of the cut-off point between pass and fail (see, e.g. Silva, McGee and Williams, 1983; Dixon, Kot and Law, 1988; Fischel et al., 1989; Walker et al., 1989; Rescorla, 1989).

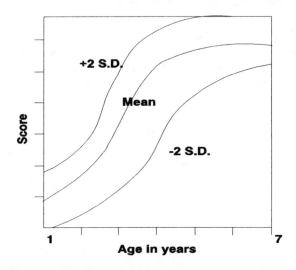

**Figure 18.3** Reynell Expressive Language Scale. A raw score of 47 is achieved by the average child at age 4 years; but by 3% of children at age 2;6 – and 3% of children do not reach this level until age 6;0.

*Performance of the Tests*

A second problem about screening is to do with the performance of the available tests. The best researched of all developmental tests, the Denver, was not originally designed to screen for language problems (Frankenburg, Chen and Thomton, 1988) and does not perform well in this regard. Other screening instruments are available, though only a few have been properly evaluated; some rely on professional assessment, others on parental report (e.g. Dale, 1989; Glascoe, 1991). It is important that a screening test should correlate well with the definitive formal assessment, in order to minimise false positives and negatives. A great deal of research effort has been devoted to the construction of screening tests, but I do not believe that the adequacy or otherwise of the tests is the major issue.

## Does Intervention Work?

A third argument against screening is that intervention does not work anyway, and therefore detection is a waste of time. While I share the critics' doubts about the value of what is currently on offer for many children, the literature does not support such a nihilistic view. Undoubtedly, a much greater proportion of the research effort should be devoted to studies of intervention; we have only to look at the papers presented for this conference to see how little interest this has attracted.

## Multiple Screening Would be Essential

The fourth serious problem about screening for language delay is that language competence changes as the child matures (e.g. Silva, 1987; Field, Fox and Radcliffe, 1990; Shapiro et al., 1990). Many speech and language therapists believe that 'delayed' children should be discovered and referred as young as possible, perhaps even before the second birthday and certainly before the third. To the extent that the process of language acquisition might be influenced by the child's early language experiences, this is a reasonable proposition. Unfortunately, the younger the child, the more difficult it is to determine which children really have a problem. Even at the age of four, it is by no means easy to make reliable predictions about outcome 18 months later. A child who is 'delayed' at age three or five is not necessarily delayed at age seven; more important, a child who is not delayed at age three may be at age five or seven. This means that several screening procedures might be needed.

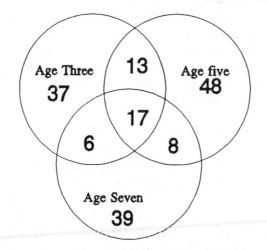

**Figure 18.4** Number of children with speech–language delay at each of three ages. Total no. = 857 (data of Silva, 1987).

## A Means of Regulating Demand

The fifth problem is that the pass–fail criteria which determine whether or not a child 'passes' a screening test are too easily manipulated, whether consciously or not, in order to regulate the number of children deemed to have a developmental problem. This phenomenon is well recognised in education (Morris, 1988), particularly in regard to resources for remedial reading. The more remedial teachers are available, the more reading retarded children will be discovered.

## The Inverse Care Law

Perhaps the most serious disadvantage of a screening procedure relates to the inverse care law: 'Those who most need professional care are least likely to access and use it'. The language-delayed children who we do not see in our child health screening clinics and who our conscientious health visitors often cannot find or visit, are probably also those who would most benefit from expert help. In everyday practice in the UK, the coverage of 3-year-olds for routine screening examinations rarely exceeds 60% and is often as low as 40%. Families living under stressful conditions have priorities that differ from those of middle-class families. That is not to say that they do not care about their children; but rather that they have other and more immediate worries than the fact that their child is slow to talk. They believe that the child will talk eventually, provided that he is not deaf or brain damaged, and the supposed links between language development and educational success are too abstract to engage their attention.

To summarise, I have argued that screening for speech and language problems would have to target all children with 'delay', since there is no simple means of screening for subgroups of delayed children; that the development of satisfactory screening tests is technically possible; but that such an approach has a number of inherent problems. What solutions can we offer to these dilemmas?

## Where do we go From Here?

Developmental screening is an idea whose time has passed. There is a period in the evolution of a nation's healthcare system when it may be valuable, after the major causes of child morbidity and mortality have been conquered but before there is widespread awareness of the serious handicapping conditions of childhood. But now we should be striving for a system which provides appropriate opportunities for all children rather than requiring us to select and label an arbitrary number of 'special needs' children. I was pleased to find this view clearly articulated by a North American writer (Ireton, 1990):

> In the future, health professionals, mental health professionals and educators may be able to collaborate to provide continuity of care, education, and support to young children and their parents in ways that will make screening... obsolete. A longitudinal, developmentally oriented care and educational system could be far superior to any cross sectional screening approach for meeting the needs of young children in general and children with special problems in particular.

In the UK, we have made a start. The Report of the Joint Working Party, 'Health For All Children' proposed that routine developmental screening examinations should be discontinued (Hall, 1991). A programme of five routine health checks was recommended; at birth, and at 2 months, 6–9 months, 18–24 months, and a preschool check at about 3;6 years. These reviews involve the skills of both doctors and health visitors. Formal screening tests are not used, but the health visitors have a detailed knowledge of child development and use this to assist parents in deciding whether their child has any particular developmental problems or needs; it is still important to ascertain whether any special educational provision might be necessary.

The time devoted to a family is governed by their needs and concerns, and staff are encouraged to use their professional judgment, in the light of parental expectations, and to apply their knowledge of local resources. They also facilitate access to services which could help high-stress families improve their skills in child care, and such families receive far more input than competent well-functioning families.

The Joint Working Party also advised that greater use should be made of the abilities of parents, relatives and other community workers such as playgroup leaders, to identify problems. The role of health professionals is to facilitate access to services whenever there is any concern, for diagnosis and management. Clearly, there is a need for better education of all professionals about child development if such a programme is to be successful; fortunately, there is now a sufficient scientific basis for the subject for this to be possible. There is an urgent need for a dialogue between health and education. Professionals working in these two giant public services meet surprisingly rarely and do not often share their rather different perceptions of the developmental needs of young children.

We need to invest in two activities; education for parents, and universal access to early educational expertise. The National Curriculum could very well integrate child care and development into the educational programme, as part of Personal, Social and Health Education, so that young people would leave school with more understanding of the needs of children and of their normal development. Individual guidance would continue to be provided where necessary by the health-visiting network, particularly for young and unsupported mothers, and by self-help projects like NewPin.

Universal nursery school education should be supported by extended day care and by reduction in school holiday breaks, so that the nurseries can provide for the single working parents who have most need of such care for their children. As soon as a child is attending nursery, nursery school or formal school, teaching staff can monitor the child's progress continuously and should have easy access to specialist advice. They would identify children with developmental difficulties and would call on the expertise of others when detailed assessment is needed. The National Curriculum concepts could be extended to provide simple language development targets, for children in the pre-school age group; the notion of helping each child to achieve a minimum standard may be easier to deal with in practice than that of screening for 'delay'. Speech and language therapists would associate themselves with the educational system rather than try to tackle the impossible task of giving individual therapy to children in community health clinics.

Such a solution would remove the need to screen and label children; it would be flexible in response to the changing needs of young children; it would devote resources to intervention instead of detection. Criterion number 9 of the Wilson and Jungner criteria states that 'the cost of case-finding should be economically balanced in relation to expenditure on medical care as a whole'.

At present, many Districts (including my own) have an expensive network of doctors and health visitors engaged in the task of case finding but the waiting list for a speech therapy assessment is about 9 months. Developmental screening has become a means of gate-keeping so that we can regulate the flow of children referred to therapists and to education at a level they can cope with. These comments are not a plea for more speech and language therapists, but for a more imaginative and rational approach to the wider problems of care for young children.

## What Would it Cost?

Can we afford it? That is a political question; the borough where my hospital is situated, Wandsworth, noted for having set the lowest poll tax in the UK, believes that it can and is about to introduce universal free nursery school education. We will wait and see what the cost may be in terms of other services lost. But if we want to achieve the best for the largest number of children, I suggest that this is the way forward.

# References

BISHOP, D.V.M. (1989). Autism, Asperger's syndrome, and semantic–pragmatic disorder: where are the boundaries? *British Journal of Disorders of Communication,* **24,** 107–121.

BISHOP, D.V.M. and ADAMS, C. (1990). A prospective study of the relationship between specific language impairment, phonological disorders and reading retardation. *Journal of Child Psychology and Psychiatry,* **31,** 1027–1050.

BUTLER, J. (1989). *Child Health Surveillance in Primary Care: a critical review.* London: HMSO.

DALE, P., BATES, E., REZNICK, S. and MORRISET, C. (1989). The validity of a parent report instrument of child language at twenty months. *Journal of Child Language,* **16,** 239–250.

DIXON, J., KOT, A. and LAW, J. (1988). Early language screening in City and Hackney: work in progress. *Child: Care, Health and Development,* **14,** 213–229.

DRILLIEN, C. and DRUMMOND, M. (1983). Developmental screening and the child with special needs. *Clinics in Developmental Medicine, Volume 86.* London: Heinemann.

FIELD, M., FOX, N. and RADCLIFFE, J. (1990). Predicting IQ change in preschoolers with developmental delays. *Journal of Developmental and Behavioral Pediatrics,* **11,** 184–189.

FISCHEL, J.E., WHITEHURST, G.J., CAULFIELD, M.B. and DEBARYSHE, B. (1989). Language growth in children with expressive language delay. *Pediatrics,* **83,** 218–227.

FRANKENBURG, W.K., CHEN, J. and THORNTON, S.M. (1988). Common pitfalls in the evaluation of developmental screening tests. *Journal of Pediatrics,* **113,** 1110–1113.

GLASCOE, F.P. (1991). Can clinical judgment detect children with speech–language problems? *Pediatrics,* **87,** 317–322.

HAGGARD, M.P. and HUGHES, E. (1991). *Screening Children's Hearing: A Review of the Literature and Implications of Otitis Media.* London: HMSO.

HALL, D.M.B., HILL, P. and ELLIMAN, D. (1990). *The Child Surveillance Handbook.* Oxford: Radcliffe.

HALL, D.M.B. (1991). *'Health For All Children', the Report of the Joint Working Party on Child Health Surveillance (2nd edn.).* Oxford: OUP.

IRETON, H. (1990). Developmental screening measures. In: Johnson, J.H. and Goldman, J. (Eds), *Developmental Assessment in Clinical Child Psychology.* New York: Pergamon.

LEONARD, L.B. (1987). Is specific language impairment a useful construct? In: Rosenburg, S. (Ed.), *Advances in Psycholinguistics, Volume 1.* Cambridge: CUP.

MORRIS, R.D. (1988). Classification of learning disabilities: Old problems and new approaches. *Journal of Consulting and Clinical Psychology,* **56,** 789–794.

RESCORLA, L. (1989). The language development survey: a screening tool for delayed language in toddlers. *Journal of Speech and Hearing Disorders,* **54,** 587–599.

SHAPIRO, B.K., PALMER, F.B., ANTELL, S., BILKER, S., ROSS A. and CAPUTE, A.J. (1990). Precursors of reading delay: neurodevelopmental milestones. *Pediatrics,* **85,** 416–420.

SILVA, P.A. (1987). Epidemiology, longitudinal course and some associated factors: an update. In: Yule, W. and Rutter, M. (Eds), *Language Development and Disorders.* Oxford: Blackwells.

SILVA, P.A., MCGEE, R. and WILLIAMS, S.M. (1983). Developmental language delay from three to seven years and its significance for low intelligence and reading difficulties at age seven. *Developmental Medicine and Child Neurology*, **25**, 83–93.

WALKER, D., GUGENHEIM, S., DOWNS, M.P. and NORTHERN, J.L. (1989). Early language milestone scale and language screening of young children. *Pediatrics*, **83**, 284–288.

WELLS, G. (1985). *Language Development in the Pre-school Years*. Cambridge: CUP.

WING, L. (1988). The continuum of autistic characteristics. In: Schopler, E. and Mesibov, G.B. (Eds), *Diagnosis and Assessment in Autism*. New York: Plenum.

# Index